Regressive Movements in Times of Emergency

Regressive Movements in Times of Emergency

The Protests against Anti-contagion Measures and Vaccination during the Covid-19 Pandemic

Donatella della Porta

Scuola Normale Superiore

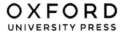

OXFORD
UNIVERSITY PRESS

Great Clarendon Street, Oxford, OX2 6DP,
United Kingdom

Oxford University Press is a department of the University of Oxford.
It furthers the University's objective of excellence in research, scholarship,
and education by publishing worldwide. Oxford is a registered trade mark of
Oxford University Press in the UK and in certain other countries

© Donatella della Porta 2023

Published in the United States of America by Oxford University Press
198 Madison Avenue, New York, NY 10016, United States of America

British Library Cataloguing in Publication Data

Data available

Library of Congress Control Number: 2023937961

ISBN 9780198884309

DOI: 10.1093/oso/9780198884309.001.0001

Printed and bound by
CPI Group (UK) Ltd, Croydon, CR0 4YY

Links to third party websites are provided by Oxford in good faith and
for information only. Oxford disclaims any responsibility for the materials
contained in any third party website referenced in this work.

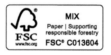

MIX
Paper | Supporting
responsible forestry
FSC
www.fsc.org   FSC® C013604

Acknowledgements

As is the case with many scientific enterprises, this book (as well as the research project that it builds upon) is also the product of a number of challenges and opportunities. Indeed, the so-called anti-vax protests were puzzling for me both as a citizen and as a scholar. Just like many friends and colleagues, I also came into contact with distant relatives who, embedded as they were in New Age or conservative Catholic milieus, had suddenly converted to conspiracy beliefs about Bill Gates putting microchips in vaccines, the World Health Organization spreading viruses (and imposing vaccination) in order to actually reduce the global population by killing millions of people, or human foetuses being used to produce anti-Covid 'serums'. What shocked me was not only the absurdity of these beliefs, but also their lack of permeability from the outside. I had previously found similar cognitive closure when studying political violence in members of underground organizations, but in those cases it often grew as a result of long-term experience in a totalitarian community, while in the case of the anti-vax activists the process seemed to take place much more swiftly, as part of vicious cycles that involved increasing levels of isolation within closed communities.

At the same time, an image began to spread in the media of an emerging social movement, hybridizing symbols and values from various, heterogeneous backgrounds that seemed to challenge some of the main theoretical assumptions in social movement studies. Presented as the result of a quite spontaneous convergence of people with different ideological backgrounds, the anti-vax protests seemed to dispense with the need for both previous networks and resources as well as certain shared normative positions. While it was clear from the very beginning that far-right activists were present at the protests, the participants also seemed to include middle-aged people with no previous activist experience. The slogans appeared to be as incoherent as the outlook of the protestors, with calls to save nature intermingled with climate change denialism or the invocation of freedom in the face of a 'sanitary dictatorship' mixed with Nazi and Fascist symbols, and national flags displayed side by side with appeals to the President of the United States, Donald Trump, to save the world.

For an empirically oriented sociologist like me, these puzzling elements called for fieldwork research; I was fortunate enough to be able to engage in this in real time. From a theoretical point of view, having worked on the progressive side of mobilizations during the pandemic, I had already developed an interest in the effects of emergency critical junctures on contentious politics. While writing the recently published *Contentious Politics in Emergency Critical Junctures. Progressive Social Movements during the Pandemic*, I had built upon social science research on collective action in times of emergency, with a particular attention on health catastrophes. In doing so, I had formed a number of reflections on eventful periods as historical moments in which agency and contingency acquire importance to a greater extent than in normal times. Studying progressive movements, I therefore developed an interest in understanding how the very same critical juncture can affect movements at different ends of the political spectrum, while also establishing some analytic tools to address these questions. Moreover, while my research to date has mainly addressed progressive movements, my understanding of regressive social movements was aided by work that I had previously carried out on the Far Right, as well as a recent publication project on the backlash (led by Karen Alter and Michael Zuern).

Research funding from the Carlo Azeglio Ciampi Institute for Advanced Studies at the Scuola Normale Superiore, as well as from the Tuscany Region, made it possible to develop parts of the empirical investigation. Following six years as the founding Dean of the Faculty of Political and Social Sciences at the Scuola Normale Superiore, a sabbatical year from 2021 to 2022 offered me some much welcome time to focus on the tasks of researching and writing. This was undertaken while generously hosted by the Center for Civil Society Research at the Social Science Center in Berlin, which offered a stimulating environment in which to advance my comparative perspective on both progressive and regressive movements during the pandemic. During this same period, I was honoured to be awarded the Research Prize of the Alexander von Humboldt Foundation and to be nominated as an International Honorary Member of the American Academy of Art and Sciences, both of which provided me with additional motivation to progress with my project.

As any scientific enterprise forms part of a wider collective effort, I wish to thank all of the colleagues and friends with whom I was able to exchange my ideas. Over the past number of years, I have discussed my data and interpretation at various conferences in Crete, Dublin, Prague, Dresden, Lisbon, Paris, Bielefeld, Berlin, and elsewhere. I would like to express my gratitude to the organizers and participants of these events for the stimulating discussions that were had. I am also grateful for the possibility to deepen my analysis during various events at the Centre on Social Movement Studies (Cosmos) in the Scuola Normale Superiore, such as those organized with Lorenzo Bosi,

Guglielmo Meardi, Mario Pianta, Hans-Jorg Trenz, and Lorenzo Zamponi, among others. I was also able to learn a great deal from other research projects I have directed at the Scuola Normale Superiore in collaboration with Chiara Milan, Carlotta Caciagli, and Giada Bonu Rosenkranz. Along with Riccardo Chesta, Daniela Chironi, and Andrea Felicetti I was involved in an empirical investigation on health movements, civic society, communication, and science during the pandemic. Anna Lavizzari has been a brilliant collaborator as part of a research project on contentious politics during the pandemic, and carried out the protest event analysis included in Chapter 2 of this volume. As this chapter builds upon our co-authored article 'Waves in Cycle: The protests against anti-contagion measures and vaccination in Covid-19 times in Italy' in *Partecipazione e Conflitto* (2022), I wish to thank the journal for the permission to refer to it. Stella Christou investigated the Greek case study, which is also addressed in this volume. Andrea Pirro helped me to update my knowledge on the Far Right. With regard to the German case study, I collaborated with Swen Hutter and Sophia Hunger as well as Edgar Grande at the Social Science Center in Berlin. I am very grateful to each and every one of them. I also wish to thank Emmet Marron for his careful language editing, Dominic Byatt at Oxford University Press for his detailed oversight of this volume, as well as the anonymous referees for their very helpful suggestions.

Contents

List of Figures

1

Regressive Movements in Times of Emergency

An Introduction

The protests against anti-contagion measures and vaccination during the Covid-19 pandemic: An introduction

Since the very beginning of the pandemic, while progressive movements mainly focused on social inequalities, often calling for investment in the public health system and vaccination for all (della Porta 2022), protests also targeted the policy measures that governments took in order to reduce contagion, such as lockdowns, mask wearing, social distancing, contact reduction, and vaccination. As early as April 2020, demonstrators called 'end the lockdown' protests in several countries. Across the United States, protesters carried posters reading, 'Your health is not more important than my liberties', 'Sacrifice the weak', 'Social distancing = Communism', and 'Muzzles are for dogs and slaves'. On 30 April 2020, heavily armed men occupied the Michigan State Capitol to protest against lockdown measures. Although less violent, protests with similar claims took place in Europe, emerging first in Germany and then spreading to other countries. After a series of smaller protests at the local level and a national demonstration on 1 August 2020, a second national protest mobilized about 30,000 protesters in Berlin on 29 August, including a group of right-wing activists that attempted to storm the national parliament (Teune 2021). In May 2020, anti-lockdown protests were organized by the UK Freedom Movement, first at Hyde Park, with a subsequent larger protest taking place in August 2020. In Italy, on 31 May 2020 a demonstration against the 'lie' of the pandemic was called in Milan by 'orange vests', led by a former Carabinieri colonel, Antonio Pappalardo, who had already become known for having led a (failed) *forconi* (pitchforks) rebellion (Gerbaudo 2020). Other protests were to follow during the years of the pandemic.

Regressive Movements in Times of Emergency. Donatella della Porta, Oxford University Press. © Donatella della Porta (2023). DOI: 10.1093/oso/9780198884309.003.0001

From the outbreak of Covid-19, these protests have received sustained attention, with both the mass media and social media focusing on the pandemic. Initial comments often pointed at the heterogeneity of the participants, who seemed to belong to different milieus, from the Far Right to New Age groups that opposed mainstream medicine and suggested alternative treatments instead. In Germany, the use of the self-definition 'Querdenker' (literally, those who think 'laterally') pointed to a critical view that rejected any distinction between left- and right-wing ideologies and rather promoted the resistance of the 'people' against an almighty, hidden 'elite', something that was also stated by protestors in other countries. Conspiracy beliefs—from the politicized QAnon and Great Replacement conspiracies widespread on the Far Right to the chemtrails and 5G theories (i.e., the fifth generation of mobile phone networks) present within the New Age milieu that promoted alternative health practices—were clearly visible in both the slogans and symbols used by the protestors. At different moments in different countries, contestation of the anti-Covid-19 measures proceeded with peaks and troughs, following the waves of contagion and the related rise in policy measures to try to curb them. These protests saw a significant increase during the vaccination campaigns; however, as the Covid-19 virus began to become endemic and widespread vaccination succeeded in reducing its lethality, they seemed to subside quite quickly.

In what follows, I will build on social movement studies in an attempt to illuminate the dynamics of these protests throughout the various steps of their emergence, growth, and decline. Referring to recent theoretical developments, this work will contribute in particular to the analysis of contentious politics during times of emergency, which are characterized by deep disruption to everyday life and rapid structural transformations in society. In order to understand how specific strains are transformed into actions, I will consider the opportunities and challenges faced by different actors in moments of intense mobilization in which various, contrasting claims are put forward. While these moments are rich in innovation, I will observe that they build upon an existing social movement infrastructure that contributes to give meaning to dissatisfaction by proposing a shared conceptualization of problems and solutions.

While it is undoubtably true that the pandemic triggered a great deal of discontent, the politicization of the grievances and related development of collective action were structured by existing material and symbolic resources that had been built in previous waves of protests around different *social movement families*, which are defined as a set of social movements that share general aims and often converge on common campaigns (della Porta and

Rucht 1995). While not exclusively, attention in social movement studies has, to date, focused particularly on the left-libertarian movement family, which is so called for its defence of social justice and collective freedoms (Kitschelt 1995). However, some research has also addressed the far-right movement family. Building upon and updating the analysis of similarities and differences in mobilization processes on the left and the right of the political spectrum, defined on the basis of the ideological positions of the actors as well as at their organizational basis, I suggest that the movement families most active during the Covid-19 pandemic can be referred to as *progressive* and *regressive*, with the organized protests against lockdowns, masks, social distancing, and vaccination forming part of the latter. These protests, I contend, did indeed develop as a reaction to perceived triggers relating to individual freedoms, and built upon the material and symbolic resources provided by a number of transformations within both the Far Right and a certain section of the New Age milieu that took part in the collective mobilization. At the same time, I will show that the anti-vax protests had an impact on both milieus, with effects in terms of further transformations.

It is important to note that in this work I am referring neither to vaccine hesitancy nor to all types of specific criticism relating to anti-contagion measures, but rather to the organized movement that emerged against those measures. While the protests addressed the entire wide range of anti-contagion measures, I will argue that the refusal to be vaccinated was at their core. The term 'anti-vax' is defined by the Cambridge Dictionary as 'used to describe a person or group that does not agree with vaccinating people (=giving them injections to prevent disease and spread and encourages opinions against vaccines)'('Anti-Vax' n.d.).[1] The anti-vaccine movement has been defined as being made up of those 'who intentionally refuse vaccines whenever possible and are often willing to express their vaccine skepticism with others' (Snow and Bernatzky 2023: 186). In order to distinguish different degrees of refusal, Ward (2016) singled out an anti-vaccine movement, marginally anti-vaccine movements, and the occasionally critical vaccine movement. Historically, there have been various waves of anti-vaccination campaigns, often located within religious groupings—beginning in the 1700s with campaigns against variolation (which involved the deliberate infection of individuals with a milder variant of the disease), and then continuing against the compulsory vaccination imposed by the British and American governments in the 1800s. In several countries, the most recent anti-vax movement developed in the late 1990s based on alleged (and fake) claims about a link between autism and

---

[1] https://dictionary.cambridge.org/dictionary/english/anti-vax (accessed 20 March 2022).

the MMR (measles, mumps, and rubella) vaccine. The analysis presented in this book will focus on the organized dimension of the opposition to anti-contagion measures, most prominently vaccination, during the Covid-19 pandemic.

In considering organized anti-vax movements, social science interpretations have mainly been focused on the macro and the micro levels of analysis. At the macro-level, anti-vax protests have been linked to broader transformations in society, such as the spread of radical forms of individualism within the liquid society, growing insecurity, and the increasing use of social media as a channel of communication, interacting with a move towards a post-truth society. The Great Regression that followed the Great Recession, with related drops in institutional trust as well as increasing attacks on civil rights, opened up political opportunities for anti-vax mobilizations with their politicization on the Far Right. This was especially visible in countries such as Brazil or the United States, where they received the explicit support of their respective heads of state, Jair Bolsonaro and Donald Trump. At the micro-level, specific psychopathologies as well as feelings of fear have been mentioned in attempting to explain the spread of conspiracy beliefs, in particular those relating to the denial of the existence of the virus and the plots linked to vaccination. What has remained less central to date is a more orthodox social movement approach, with a focus on the meso level, which might explain how grievances are mobilized into collective action. In order to fill this gap, the analysis carried out here will build on some of the main concepts in social movement studies in order to better understand some characteristics of the anti-vax protests, such as mobilized organizational resources, repertoires of action, and collective framing.

It is undoubtedly important to consider general societal trends and individual propensities when attempting to explain anti-vax protests. Indeed, in social movement studies, political and discursive opportunities have been central concepts for understanding the development of social movements, while individual choices have been analysed in attempting to explain paths of recruitment and sustained commitment. As social movement studies suggest, however, in order to connect social structure and individual grievances to collective action, one needs to investigate the ways in which actors express their claims, how they organize, and how they frame their own action. Macro trends are, in fact, mediated by the dynamics of the protest waves, with their complex repertoires of action, organizational models, and collective framing. Thus, in order to relate structural conditions and individual grievances to collective action, one needs to investigate the ways in which actors express their claims, how they organize themselves, and how they frame their own actions.

Moreover, this evolution is also affected by the main actors and milieus that take part in these protests, in ways that still need to be analysed.

Building upon social movement studies, the research presented here looks, then, at how the anti-vax protests developed. The remainder of this introductory chapter will present the main subject of the analysis. Firstly, it will introduce the main tenets for the conceptualization of anti-vax protests as regressive movements in emergency critical junctures. Following this, it will locate the Covid-19 pandemic within general trends in societal developments, with a particular focus on the spread of individualist values and the growth of societal fragmentation. Then, linking these trends with the specific mobilization against the anti-contagion policy measures, it will address the spread of conspiracy theories as well as the emergence of a political backlash, with particular attention paid to the evolution in the Far Right, through ultra-nationalist and anti-gender frames. It will then move on to outline how social movement studies might contribute to our understanding of contentious politics during the pandemic by connecting the meso with both the macro and micro levels of analysis. It will conclude with a presentation of the research design of the empirical analysis and an outline of the structure of the volume.

Regressive movements in emergency critical junctures

Building on my recent work on social movements, in this volume I aim to locate the anti-vax protests within a theoretical reflection on social movements during times of crisis. The Covid-19 crisis can be defined as an *emergency critical juncture*, characterized by a sudden rupture produced by a global catastrophic event, triggered by an airborne, highly contagious virus, which quickly prompted economic, social, and political crises (della Porta 2022). In general, social movements can produce, or at least adapt to, what neo-institutionalists call critical junctures. These are defined as '(1) a major episode of institutional innovation, (2) occurring in distinct ways, (3) and generating an enduring legacy' (Collier and Munck 2017: 2). In contrast to normal periods, critical junctures are often linked to periods of 'crisis or strain that existing policies and institutions are ill-suited to resolve' (Roberts 2015: 65).

In social movement studies, attention has turned anew to the role of contentious politics in exceptional periods, when 'the accepted norms of behaviour, the ones that guide behaviours in everyday, institutionalized, normal, quotidian activities, don't apply because of unusual or atypical social contexts: a catastrophe, a suddenly imposed grievance, a moral shock, a disaster' (Johnston 2018: 8). Critical events alter both the environmental conditions and our perceptions of them, increasing the potential for coalition but also for division. In general, extraordinary challenges have 'profound effects on the structuring of strategic action fields across society' by undermining 'all kinds of linkages in society and make it difficult for groups to reproduce their power' (Fligstein and McAdam 2012: 101). At the same time, dramatic disruptions prompt the 'attribution of new opportunities and threats leading to the appropriation or creation of new organizational vehicles for the purpose of engaging in innovative, contentious interaction with other field actors' (ibid.). However, as several studies on such critical moments have indicated (e.g., Tarrow 1994), the specific balance of threats and opportunities that emerge for contentious politics in extraordinary periods varies, as it is influenced by the general social and political conditions that preceded it but also by the nature of the disruption itself. These times are in general under-structured and unpredictable, and therefore open to contingency and enhanced agency being influenced by the unfolding of social movements.

The Covid-19 pandemic can be considered a critical moment as it triggered a sudden and dramatic emergency that has deeply affected peoples' lives. Global threats, such as the Covid-19 pandemic, act as critical junctures that, however, produce different effects on different movements. While at its onset lockdown policies constrained collective action in the street, protests subsequently sprang up, triggered by severe crises that accompanied the spread of the virus.

As I have noted in my previous research on progressive social movements (della Porta 2022), social movements studies have occasionally addressed moments of emergency including health crises, natural disasters, deep economic recessions, and wars, suggesting that these critical periods are ripe with contentious politics, occurring in different forms and with diverse aims. Moments of intense crisis often intensify calls for rights by disrupting the quotidian and triggering discontent, but also by creating the expectation that sacrifices have to be compensated by tangible recognition of belonging to a community of destiny (Tilly 1992: 10). Even before the onset of the current pandemic, the recent past had been defined as a momentous period: the terms 'the great transformation', 'the great recession' as well as 'the great regression' have frequently been used as short-hands to define the period following the financial breakdown of 2008 that triggered the sizeable mobilization of so called 'movements of the crises' (della Porta and Mattoni 2014; della Porta 2015). In this context, researchers have increasingly addressed protests as transformative events that react to sudden challenges but that also themselves trigger change (della Porta 2020). Indeed, as we will see, the anti-vax protests

spread as the initial events were emulated by emerging groupings, which connected them to different grievances. New groups were formed to coordinate
the protest, interacting with existing organizations. A repertoire of action
also developed that involved copycat effects. Furthermore, over time conspiracy visions spread, with various groupings converging on a dichotomic
vision that viewed events through the prism of a battle between absolute good
and evil. Eventually, this conspiracy thinking tended to produce sectarian
dynamics, which only led to anti-vax groups becoming even more isolated.

All of this took place in an emergency situation, which triggered frustration as a result of the rapid and dramatic transformation in everyday life. It
is undoubtable that emergency periods require a careful assessment of the
trade-off between different rights and liberties. As Baldwin (Baldwin 2005:
247) noted in a comparative analysis of health policies during the Aids pandemic, 'attempts to curtail epidemics raise—in the guise of public health—the
most enduring political dilemma: how to reconcile the individual's claim to
autonomy and liberty with the community's concern with safety .... How
are individual rights and the public good pursued simultaneously?'. We can
add here that exceptional circumstances, such as global pandemics, create
dilemmas not only between individual liberties and public security, but also
between health protection and other social rights, since lockdown measures
halt or dramatically reduce access to social or educational public services as
well as other services, including public transport.

During the Covid-19 crisis, these dilemmas have been apparent as states of
emergency have been called in different forms by different countries. Indeed,
the pandemic has been considered 'a social and economic shock as well as
a political crisis and a psychological trauma. There was an abrupt end to
mobility as, one by one, states imposed lockdowns and quarantines with
the result that normal life ceased ... What at first seemed possible only in
a dictatorship became an increasingly accepted way to respond to the danger
posed by the coronavirus' (Delanty 2021: 1). While states of emergency are
contemplated in democratic regimes in order to address various types of disasters, there is no doubt that they affect citizens' rights, reducing the checks
and balances on institutions as well as the capacity of citizens to hold their
governments accountable. As governance in emergencies tends to be informal and unaccountable, exceptional powers break with procedural rules,
with the suspension of some rights and a centralization of decision-making.
Paradoxically, 'While emergency rule entails frenetic decision making, its
decisions are rationalized as unchosen and unavoidable in substance and timing' (White 2021: 85). Given that the most important decisions are taken in
haste, emergencies also increase discretion, due to a lack of clarity about the

limits and the implications of the decisions taken (ibid.: 81). As Scheppele (2010: 133–4) has synthetized, emergency scripts involve (i) executive centralization, with a decline in the power of the parliament; (ii) militarization, with the military positioned as key respondent to the threat; (iii) procedural shortcuts, as procedural checks are bypassed; (iv) a ban on demonstrations, with restrictions on freedom of movement; (v) constraints on freedom of speech, with censorship and criminalization; and (vi) decreasing transparency, with governmental action blanketed in secrecy as well as increasing surveillance up to and including anticipatory violence against opponents. In the case of the Covid-19 pandemic, attempts have been made to address the crisis through emergency measures that have dramatically constrained rights of movement, expatriation, assembly, speech, and information. While this has happened to different degrees in different regimes—with more drastic and arbitrary constraints in authoritarian regimes—the very presence of an emergency has undoubtedly affected the functioning of public institutions at all territorial levels as well as on a worldwide scale.

A further aspect that has been highlighted by the Covid-19 crisis is the fact that emergencies affect not only civil rights, but also social rights, as they magnify the effects of the unequal distribution of resources within and across countries. Social protection is especially at stake as living conditions related to core social rights (such as health, work, housing, and education) are jeopardized by exceptional circumstances. As is the case during war, catastrophes, or deep economic depressions, the disruption of everyday life during pandemics hits some sections of the population especially hard, increasing class, gender, generational, and ethnic inequalities. While a disruption of everyday life has been a common experience worldwide during the Covid-19 pandemic, the degree of suffering has been unquestionably influenced by pre-existing conditions in terms of social rights. The virus has especially highlighted the lethal consequences of differential access to public health care, revealing the 'weakness of state capacity—underfunded, part-privatized and underprepared health systems' (White 2021: 77). As a result, while the Covid-19 pandemic was initially presented as having a levelling effect, 'as the pathogen infects human beings indiscriminately of social status and the containment measures disrupted the economic engines of whole national economies, the public health crisis in fact laid bare existing inequalities and deepened them farther' (Azmanova 2021: 244). It must be noted that health crises also have a disruptive effect on solidarity, especially as contagious diseases are more likely to spread suspicion among members of the community, thus reducing resilience. Although the attribution of personal similarity to the victims can increase compassion, when this similarity is denied, the victims are often blamed, rumours are spread, and moral panics are frequently triggered. Indeed, the higher the mortality rate of a contagious disease, the fear of others and the level of scapegoating, the more interpersonal trust breaks down.

The disruption caused to existing links and routines by emergency critical junctures triggers contentious politics, both progressive and regressive in nature. While I recognize that progress is a contested term (Allen 2016), I have defined as *progressive* those social movements that share a combined attention to social justice and positive freedom with the so-called left-libertarian movement family of the past (della Porta and Rucht 1995; della Porta 2020). Progress is thus understood as:

> the liberation (or 'emancipation') of collectivities (for example: citizens, classes, nations, minorities, income categories, even mankind), be it the liberation from want, ignorance, exploitative relations, or the freedom of such collectives to govern themselves autonomously, that is, without being dependent upon or controlled by others. Furthermore, the freedom that results from liberation applies equally to all, with equality serving as a criterion to make sure that liberation does not in fact become a mere privilege of particular social categories.
>
> **(Offe 2011: 79–80)**

Thus, progressive movements are those that raise claims for a broader inclusion of citizens and a reduced domination both within and across national borders (Ypi 2012). In doing so, they endorse equality as the core value of the Left (Bobbio 1997).

On the opposite side, some movements can be conceptualized as *regressive* actors, when they aim at returning to a previous and less inclusive, or worse, state or way of behaving, which can also be defined as retrograde (aimed at returning to old and worse conditions) or reactionary (i.e., opposed to political and social change).[2] The Great Recession of the early 2010s has been connected with a Great Regression in terms of civil and political rights. In relation to this, Karen Alter and Michael Zürn (2020: 4) have defined backlash politics as 'a particular form of political contestation with a retrograde objective as well as extraordinary goals or tactics that has reached the threshold level of entering public discourse'. Social movement studies have looked at movements with *retrograde objectives*—defined

---

[2] 'Regressive' definition in the Cambridge English Dictionary, https://dictionary.cambridge.org/dictionary/english/regressive (accessed 20 March 2022); 'retrograde' definition in the Cambridge English Dictionary, https://dictionary.cambridge.org/dictionary/english/retrograde (accessed 20 March 2022); 'reactionary' definition in the Cambridge English Dictionary, https://dictionary.cambridge.org/dictionary/english/reactionary (accessed 20 March 2022).

as backward-looking moves—especially in the empirical research on the far-right movements that have been considered as collective actors aiming for the reversal of the extension of rights in the name of former privileges.

Inequality (with related calls for exclusion) is considered to be a main value for the Right. In Bobbio's (1997: 59) words, in order to distinguish the Left from the Right, 'As the founding principle, equality is the only criterion that withstands the test of time, and resists the steady breakdown to which the other criteria have been subjected ... the criterion most frequently used to distinguish between the left and the right is the attitude of real people in society to the ideal of equality.' In addition, traditions play an important role in defining the Right in contrast to the Left, which calls instead for emancipation (Laponce 1981). So, 'the right-winger is primarily concerned with safeguarding tradition, and the left-winger on the other hand wishes, above everything else, to liberate his fellow human beings from the chains imposed on them by the privileges of race, class, rank, etc' (Cofrancesco 1981: 34). Together with equality versus inequality and tradition versus emancipation, the opposition between progressive and regressive movements can be defined by the privilege given to social responsibility versus personal achievement, collectivism versus individualism, collective freedoms versus individual freedom, horizontality versus hierarchy, the future versus the past.

During the pandemic, as progressive social movements mobilized in defence of what they defined as measures of solidarity with the weakest sections of the population, regressive actors contested lockdowns and hygiene measures (such as the wearing of face masks) as well as vaccination, in a narrative that, as outlined above, privileged individual freedoms over the protection of society as a whole. As I will argue in the following chapters, the anti-vax protests were regressive in nature, being promoted and carried out by a coalition of (mainly far-right) groups that embraced extreme forms of individualism, called for a return to 'natural laws' against the state and converged on conspiracy theories.

Liquid modernity, fragmented societies

When explaining both progressive and regressive types of contentious politics, the challenges of a pandemic such as Covid-19 must be read within some general societal trends. Thus, overall, the anti-vax protests can be understood as embedded in broad transformations—from a liquid society to post-democratic developments—which were themselves impacted by the pandemic and its specific characteristics.

First and foremost, the emergency critical juncture developed within what has been defined as part of the social dimension of neoliberal capitalism: a push not only for a free market approach against social protection, but also for individual freedom over security. Influentially, Zygmunt Bauman has defined a trend towards *liquid modernity* as characterized by insecurity and flexibility. In his view, postmodern men and women have 'exchanged a portion of their possibilities of security for a portion of happiness. The discontents of modernity arose from a kind of security that tolerated too little freedom in the pursuit of individual happiness. The discontents of post-modernity arise from a kind of freedom of pleasure-seeking which tolerate too little individual security' (Bauman 1997: 3). If Fordism represented the solid phase of modernity, consisting of law and routine (Bauman 2000: 63) as the lives of individuals were mainly organized around their role as producers, in liquid modernity the lives of consumers are instead dominated by seduction and volatile desires (ibid.: 76). The self-assertion of the individual goes hand-in-hand with a denial of society: 'To put in a nutshell, "individualization" consists of transforming human "identity" from a "given" into a "task"' (ibid.: 31). So, 'Modernity replaces the heteronomic determination of social standing with compulsive, and obligatory self-determination' (ibid.: 32). In this new context, collective identities are considered as difficult to develop, since individualism wins over collectivity (ibid.: 22). Most importantly, these developments imply the spread of fear, which is no longer managed through state intervention or long-term involvement in the Fordist factory but rather fuelled by deregulation-cum-individualization (ibid.: 67).

The spread of individualistic views has also been connected to a number of general transformations in the relationship between science, politics, the market, and public opinion that also affect and are affected by the pandemic. A participatory challenge to expertise has been linked to long-term developments in the cultural politics of knowledge, including 'the decline of what might be called epistemic deference; the long-standing suspicion of insular forms of expert judgment; the valorization of various forms of lay expertise; and the growing sense—especially in health and lifestyle domains—that people must educate themselves and take responsibility for arbitrating between competing expert claims' (Brubaker 2020: 78).

Of particular relevance for the understanding of the anti-vax protests, researchers have noted the danger of a politicization of science related to the use of scientists as a main source of information. Although scientists were generally found to be more trusted than politicians, and therefore better positioned to convince citizens to comply with anti-contagion regulations (Farjam et al. 2021), the overexposure of experts has also been shown to have negative effects on the communication process. Broadly speaking, when scientists communicate directly with the public about health risks, this has the potential to trigger mistrust in scientists due to the fact that 'If individuals come to see a scientist as political in their orientation, it may shape their perceptions of the scientist's credibility' (Vraga et al. 2018: 2).[3]

During the pandemic, many of the abovementioned phenomena played a role in scientific controversies on the characteristics of the virus and related preventive measures that were broadly reported in the media. The overexposure of certain scientists in the media triggered a spectacularization and polarization of the scientific debate, thus politicizing the scientific sphere, and leading to the risk of a delegitimization of scientific knowledge. It has been noted that 'Distrust in science and technology moves into the spotlight in a climate of growing understanding about the political nature of science, supplanting a view of the scientific sphere as immune from public debate and the presentation of different truth claims' (Alteri et al. 2021: 13).

The politicization of science, along with the related scientization of politics (Eyal 2019) has been considered a particular challenge of the pandemic, at a time when expertise is all the more needed in order to legitimize political decisions and have a significant direct impact on citizens. As Brubaker (2020: 75) has noted:

> it's no surprise that expertise would come under attack. The influence of epidemiologists has indeed been truly unprecedented. Never before, arguably, has so narrow a network of experts exerted so decisive and so incalculably far reaching an effect on the course of world events, upending the lives of billions and plunging the world economy into its deepest crisis since the Great Depression.

A further factor cited as fuelling mistrust in science is digital hyperconnectivity, which greatly increased not only the visibility of experts but also the availability of expertise, through easy access to databases and research findings. As a consequence, as experts advise governments and address the public, 'expert opinions, expert models and projections, expert research, and expertise-relevant data are more accessible and more abundant than ever. ... Their views, along with journalists' simplifying accounts of those views, have then been recirculated at high velocity—though often of course in fragmented and distorted form—by legions of digitally active lay users' (ibid.: 77). The spreading awareness of the relative, provisional, and imperfect nature of scientific results beyond expert circles contributed to increasing mistrust in

---

[3] There is also a particular tendency for mistrust in official science to increase when the information provided by scientists is incongruent with personal beliefs, a factor which pushes individuals to discredit scientists by attributing specific political motives to them (Vraga et al. 2018).

science in some milieus. This was particularly problematic in a situation in which the opinions of experts were presented as being most relevant for their impact on everyday life. Therefore, citizens found themselves 'direct participants in the tortuous, provisional, uncertain and fallible world of the scientific process, while scientists are cast in a public role, communicating their ideas to a wide audience and showcasing their disagreements and conflicts, removing the veil of objectivity and infallibility' (Alteri et al. 2021: 9). While there was widespread trust in science among the majority of citizens, there also seems to have been a growth of mistrust at the margins.[4]

At the same time, the abundance of expertise and the ease with which it could be accessed increased the impression that large disagreements were taking place, which was further compounded by the diffusion of semi-expert and quasi-expert opinions. A large amount of contradictory information circulated in a complex communication system. When considering the dynamics of the pandemic crisis, links have been drawn between a retrenchment of the public sphere and the ongoing transformation of the communication process, in which there is increasing conglomerate control of both mainstream media and social media, with parallel trends of scandalization and the spreading of fake news, in what has been termed the post-truth society. With an overabundance of not only facts but also rumours and speculation, disinformation spreads with attempts 'to deliberately mislead others for strategic or, perhaps, pathological purposes, through a systematic, intentional disruption of authoritative information flows' (Harsin 2020: 1061). The effects of this process include increasing uncertainty and anxiety, which may be harmful to the physical and mental health of certain individuals (WHO 2020).

Digital media, in particular, have been considered as more prone to the spread of disinformation, given the fact that their communicative dynamics promote disintermediation. Due to this, users are more and more exposed to contradictory content produced by different sources and distributed in fragmented and anonymized forms, while social media algorithms create echo chambers (e.g. Alteri et al. 2021: 17). Overall, online communication has contributed to the spread of fake news, instilling it with populist and anti-establishment tones (Boberg et al. 2020: 17).

---

[4] For instance, in Germany, according to the Science Barometer (2021), while the percentage of those who either 'completely' or 'somewhat' trusted science and research increased during the pandemic to 61% (from about 50% in the previous year), and as much as 79% trusted doctors and medical staff, 13% still stated that there is 'no evidence that Corona exists', 26% that 'the pandemic is being made into a bigger thing than it actually is' and a relatively high 39% believed that 'scientists don't tell us everything they know about the coronavirus' (for more see, https://www.wissenschaft-im-dialog.de/fileadmin/user_upload/Projekte/Wissenschaftsbarometer/Dokumente_21/EN/WiD_sciencebarometer_2021_brochure_web.pdf).

More generally, liquid culture has been related to populist trends, especially to related mistrust of various types of institutions. Social science approaches to populism have connected its spread to institutional mistrust, the rejection of expert knowledge, and the search for simplistic answers. Generally speaking, there has been an expectation among some that the emergence of the pandemic might prove unfavourable for populists (Watkins 2020) by instead fuelling support for responsible and rational anti-populist politicians, who have been contrasted with irrational and irresponsible populist voices (Galanopoulos and Venizelos 2022). At the same time, however, the pandemic and the various lockdowns may have increased fear and triggered the diffusion of a populist mood among substantial parts of the population as far as 'they have heightened distrust of expertise, exacerbated antipathy to intrusive government regulation, and amplified skepticism toward elite overprotectiveness. Critics of Corona restrictions have sought to bring together these forms of protopopulist discontent in a counter-narrative according to which misguided and out-of-touch experts, power-hungry regulators, and excessively risk-averse elites have combined to wreck the economy, destroy livelihoods, and trample on liberties' (Brubaker 2020: 82). In fact, mistrust in politicians, the media, and science has been connected to anti-vax positions and a lack of compliance with policies aimed at containing the contageon (Bargain and Aminjonov 2020; Bicchieri et al. 2020; Brodeur, Grigoryeva, and Kattan 2021).

As we will see, the spread of fear has been stimulated by the use of conspiracy beliefs by political entrepreneurs, which have promoted a dichotomized view of absolute evil against absolute good. Rather than a critical approach to science based on an openness to the gathering of new knowledge on a new virus, anti-vax organizations have instead promoted fake news—often masked as alternative scientific evidence.

Contention in health crises

In this context, emergency critical junctures are influenced by the specific characteristics of the exceptional circumstances that triggered the crisis (Quarantelli and Dynes 1977; Tierney 2019). Although the disruption of everyday life fuels frustration and outrage, the development of a collective response is heavily affected by the ways in which a problem (in this case a crisis) is framed (Rao and Greve 2017). As the narrative of an emergency develops during the events, social movements have the potential to influence the perceptions of its causes and consequences (Kreuder-Sonnen 2019).

Research on health crises has indicated that contagious diseases are particularly likely to cause suspicion to spread among members of the community, thus reducing resilience. While attribution of personal similarity to the victims can increase compassion, when similarity is denied, victims are easily blamed. In general, the outbreak of contagious diseases leads to the blaming of the infected or social groups considered to be the culprit (Rao and Greve 2017), with a frequent spread of rumours and the triggering of moral panics. As a matter of fact, the higher the mortality rate of a contagious disease, the higher the chance that others are feared and scapegoated, while interpersonal trust breaks down (ibid.). Airborne infectious diseases have especially highlighted the fragility of individuals and collectives (Delanty 2021). Indeed, historical analyses have pointed to the impact of plagues on societal evolution (Turner 2021), highlighting the capacity of microscopic viruses to trigger macroscopical changes (McNeill 1977; Snowden 2020). Other studies have also shown how the cognitive assessment of various health crises influenced their effects (Rosenberg 1989), as plagues have prompted the search for meaningful (religious or secular) interpretations (Turner 2021).

Historically speaking there have been shifts in how contagion has been defined as well as the approach taken to tackling health crises. During the Middle Ages, there was a conception of contagion being caused by infectious agents, with quarantine employed as a remedy. In the nineteenth century, illnesses were attributed to unhealthy environments and sanitation became the main method to tackle their spread. The current conception of illness points instead to personal dispositions, with appeals to discourage unhealthy habits and encourage healthy ones, entailing 'an individualization of public health as the new scientific knowledge made individual hygiene focal' (Kleres 2018: 28). Adding weight to the significance of individual behaviour and personal responsibility, medical knowledge has attributed obesity, heart diseases, or certain cancers to poor diet, tobacco use, alcohol consumption, insufficient physical exercise, etc. Increasingly, voluntary changes in individual behaviour became central to public health as a democratic ethos of good citizens included desirable health behaviour (Baldwin 2005: 15), reducing the consideration of the impact of the social context on the spread of diseases. As noted in the social construction of mental illness (Crossley 2006), epidemiological developments strengthened this individualization, something that has also been a dominant factor in the approaches taken to the Covid-19 pandemic.

Against a mainstream vision of individual responsibility, progressive social movements have pointed to collective responsibility, singling out contextual conditions linked to intersectional inequalities as having deadly effects (della Porta 2022). They have criticized the neoliberal order for the cuts in public health as well as the many inequalities that have increased the cost of the pandemic in terms of lives lost. Regressive movements have instead stressed unconstrained individual freedom, pitting healthy individuals against weaker ones. The pandemic crisis has seen a re-emergence in the public debate of the vision of individual responsibility, particularly in relation to the higher risk posed by the disease to some categories of patients, often defined as overweight individuals, those who travel frequently or those younger sections of society that pay less attention to public health regulations. The visible unequal exposure to the virus prompts solidarity reactions among progressive movements and, instead, victimization of the vulnerable people as responsible for their suffering by regressive movements. As noted in relation to the United States, but valid also elsewhere:

> the widely publicized disproportionate vulnerability of African Americans, Latinos, and Native Americans, of the urban poor, of the incarcerated, and of immigrant workers in meatpacking plants may reinforce the tacit or explicit sense, on the part of many residents of low-prevalence areas, that this is not 'their' pandemic, but one that afflicts others. Anti-lockdown protesters could easily draw, at least implicitly, on the longstanding and of course deeply racialized populist trope that contrasts the morally, politically, and even biomedically healthy 'heartland'—the 'real' America of locally rooted communities and virtuous, hard-working ordinary citizens—with the big cities, seen as sites of corruption, criminality, and disease, and understood as dominated by liberal cosmopolitan elites on the one hand and by racial, ethnic, religious, sexual, and gender minorities on the other.
>
> **(Brubaker 2020: 75–6)**

Indeed, in previous waves of protest against vaccination individualistic values had already been singled out as being widespread among anti-vax parents, many of whom had high social and educational levels and often lived in wealthy areas (Smith, Chu, and Barker 2004; Reich 2014; Gesser-Edelsburg, Shir-Raz, and Green 2016; Grignolio 2016; Anello et al. 2017). Research carried out on mobilizations against vaccination in Italy in 2017 pointed to the over representation of well-educated, middle-class activists who stated that their decisions were influenced by personal research on the topic, thus demonstrating a critical, but not sceptical, attitude towards science, albeit with a significant mistrust of mainstream medicine. Broadly disinterested in politics (with about 20% near to the Left and about 10% near to the Right, and the vast majority refusing to locate themselves on the Left–Right axis), these anti-vax parents expressed widespread support for alternative lifestyles, especially in terms of health and education (Lello 2020).

In addition to the wider question of mistrust in science, researchers have also pointed to anti-vax positions being fuelled by individualistic attitudes towards medicine and health issues that are associated with neoliberalism. More specifically, neoliberalism has been connected to a belief in the market and the individual responsibility of an entrepreneurial subject over collective well-being. Research on parents who had chosen not to vaccinate their children has noted that,

> several indicated that they 'cared only for their own children' whom they believed would be harmed by vaccination, and 2) several questioned the validity of vaccine research on grounds that 'they (as parents) were better able to care for their children and make better choices than the so-called experts'. Good parenting was then considered as bringing about a rejection of vaccination on the basis of the consumer's search for information and rejection instead for state intervention.
>
> **(Sanders and Burnett 2019: 152)**

In this perspective, the calls for freedom of choice are linked to a generalized rejection of state authority in the name of personal interests. Vaccination hesitancy thus builds upon neoliberal individualism given 'the denial of the social contract in favor of individual pursuits and in direct rejection of public health as a collective and worthwhile endeavor, ... the dismissal of community welfare in favor of the pursuit of individual prosperity ... the individualistic understandings of health and the public (and) the rejection of state authority' (ibid.).

I will suggest that this individualist trend combined with easy access to unselected information contributed to the spread of mistrust in scientific evidence. Contrary to their assertions of holding healthy critical attitudes, the promoters and followers of anti-vax views ended up spreading fake news and conspiracy theories. Individualism also impacted on the organization model employed, with a reliance on crowdsourcing and a failure to develop long terms structures.

Spreading fear: Conspiracy theories during the pandemic

A specific development from the growing mistrust in science, as well as individualization processes described above, is the diffusion of conspiracy theories, usually defined as singling out an evil group, operating in secrecy, and trying to acquire total power (Butter 2021). While also pointing at the risk of dismissing any social critique as conspiracy, scholars have tried to under-stand the conditions under which conspiracy theories emerge and spread (Fassin 2021). In addressing the puzzle of the recurring spread of conspir-acy beliefs even in advanced democracies and modern society,[5] sociological analysis has referred to a number of characteristics of postmodern society which include the fact that 'a hyper-connected social environment in which all sorts of knowledge and information becomes accessible, with a growing level of cognitive and educational standards, instead of spreading an enlight-ened view on reality and reducing the appeal of unprovable conjectures, has on the contrary pandered to—if not fostered—the predispositions to elabo-rate and disseminate self-made truths' (Mancosu, Vassallo, and Vezzoni 2017: 329). One of the main sets of explanations for the emergence of anti-vax protests considered the spread of conspiracy theories in terms of their causes, dynamics, and consequences.

Conspiracy theories have been defined on the basis of four common char-acteristics: 'the world or an event is held to be not as it seems; there is believed to be a cover-up by powerful others; the theory is accepted only by a minority; and the theory is unsupported by evidence' (Freeman et al. 2020: 1). Based as they are on conjectures, which are rejected by the scientific community, conspiracies:

> ascribe to particular agents (usually defined as conspirators) an extraordinary capacity to influence personal and collective decisions, to forecast the conse-quences of their actions, to maintain secrecy about their strategies, and to coor-dinate themselves in a way that goes well beyond what is realistic in an open society. They tend to assume that complex social phenomena are intentionally orchestrated by hyper-rational and omnipotent collective actors.
>
> **(Mancosu, Vassallo, and Vezzoni 2017: 327)**

According to psychological analyses, a conspiracy mentality interacts with a mistrusting mindset, fuelled by perceived vulnerability, low self-esteem, poorer psychological well-being, powerlessness, anger, and a sense of assail-ment. A situation of perceived danger fuels this process. Especially, 'A mistrusting mind-set—a defensive response of wariness—will occur when there is perceived vulnerability and a sense of assailment' (Freeman et al. 2020: 2). It has been argued that conspiracy beliefs can provide the individual

---

[5] Research in Italy has revealed that, in 2016, about half of the respondents in a representative sample considered that at least one of the four conspiracy theories put to them by researchers were plausible (Mancosu, Vassallo, and Vezzoni 2017). Similarly, in England, about half of the population showed some degree of endorsement for conspiracy ideas (Freeman et al. 2022).

believer with benefits in the short term, by reducing uncertainty and increasing a sense of control, which is linked to entering into contact (mainly online) with other people with similar mindsets and having the impression that they are accessing privileged information. Indeed, a conspiracy 'is a narrative that binds fear, excessive demands and powerlessness and gives space to the (regressive) desire to live in a world perceived as controllable or a reconciled (primordial) state with nature' (Schließler, Hellweg, and Decker 2020: 283). More widely, narcissistic gratification has been mentioned as a motivating factor, as:

> being the bearer of knowledge about secret conspiracies and systems of power, and the feeling of having access to destiny or a divine nature, make it possible to see oneself as part of an elite that—in contrast to the 'sleeping' masses—is 'awakened'. In this way, the insult that is regularly produced in a capitalist society is cushioned by the narcissistic exaggeration of one's own group of the 'awakened' or 'in the know'.
>
> (ibid.)

In a vicious cycle, conspiracy mentalities tend to cumulate, as believing in a conspiracy increases the chances of also endorsing other conspiracies (Freeman et al. 2020). In fact, conspiracy theories have been found to spread especially swiftly during critical moments (e.g., in the United States during the Cold War and McCarthyism).

During the pandemic, specific conspiracies about the virus and vaccination have been linked to other longstanding conspiracy beliefs that have been traditionally widespread against certain specific social, ethnic, or even political groups, combining fake news on vaccines with attacks against generically defined global elites, as well as the citizens who obey their orders. In particular, coronavirus conspiracy theories have ascribed malevolent intent to certain individuals, groups, and organizations, applying pre-existing prejudices to new situations. In these narratives, sometimes contradictory conspiracy statements have been connected together by mistrust in institutions and experts as well as the endorsement of other conspiracy beliefs such as those denying climate change or the assumed plot to substitute the white, Christian race with Muslims and migrants of colour, but also those claiming that chemical trails and 5G equipment are being used in a plot to control citizens or even to kill many of them in order to reduce overpopulation (Schließler, Hellweg, and Decker 2020).

What is more, the pandemic has been framed within broadly politicized conspiracy theories that consider cosmopolitan and progressive elites to be plotting against humanity. In this sense, one conspiracy theory that has been found to be particularly widespread during the pandemic is QAnon, which builds upon anti-Semitic, racist, and anti-scientific frames and connects them with fake news relating to the virus. As summarized by Rafael (2021),

> This conspiracy narrative, originally centred on Donald Trump as a saviour in the fight against evil, AKA 'the elites', with explicit anti-Semitic elements (including paedophile elites who drink children's blood), was created in the USA in 2017. An anonymous 4chan account, 'Q', claimed to be an informant from the inner-most circles of the White House and provided his followers with mysteriously incomprehensible, but very meaningful short statements—known to the fans as 'Q-Drops'—which could almost be described as clickbait for the conspiracy indus-try ('Do you feel a plot twist coming?'). Again and again, Q urged followers to wake up, think for themselves and participate. This technique brought believers to common exegesis, to a collective interpretation, welding them together to form a community—which is also reflected in the slogan 'WWG1WGA' ('Where we go one, we go all').

The QAnon conspiracy had already begun to spread to other English-speaking countries before the pandemic (in the United Kingdom it was linked to the activity of Brexit activists) and then to Germany and the rest of Europe. Endorsed by many Republicans in the US—including Donald Trump and his family—in Western Europe it was propagated through anti-EU, Islamophobic, populist-right and far-right channels which 'have enriched the antisemitic and anti-establishment narratives of the ideology with their own anti-government and anti-lockdown narratives' (ibid.). Indeed, many anti-vax groups have recycled parts of the QAnon conspiracy, such as the involvement of global elites in crimes of paedophilia, to attack policies aimed at reducing the spread of Covid-19. In a similar vein, conspiracy beliefs con-sidered cosmopolitan elites as plotting a 'Great Replacement' of the original white, Christian race in the Western world with migrants of colour and Muslims. During the pandemic, various versions of conspiracy theories also circulated on Facebook, including the idea that Bill Gates was behind the global spread of Covid-19 or the assumption that the virus had been inten-tionally leaked from a chemical laboratory in Wuhan (Boberg et al. 2020: 16).[6]

---

[6] In England, for instance, almost half of participants in a study believed that the 'Coronavirus is a bioweapon developed by China to destroy the West' and about 20 per cent that 'Jews have created the virus to collapse the economy for financial gain' (Freeman et al. 2022).

When addressing the characteristics of the anti-vax protests, I will suggest that some conspiracy theories fuelled shared visions of the virus and of vaccines in variegated organizational networks. The individual tendency of conspiracy believers to combine a range of conspiracy views helped the merging of conspiracies that were especially widespread in the Far Right, in particular QAnon and the Great Replacement, with those relating to 5G technology and the so-called chemical trails as instruments of control present in the New Age milieu as well as the conspiracy belief that foetuses were used to produce vaccines that was sponsored by anti-gender groups.

The backlash, the Far Right, and the pandemic

Conspiracy theories easily spread in liquid times, especially when political entrepreneurs exploit the subjective predispositions of individuals towards believing in them in order to use latent anti-establishment attitudes for their own purposes. If we look at the political system, initial research has often pointed to the role played by far-right actors in supporting anti-vax protests. Indeed, the emergency critical juncture presented by the Covid-19 pandemic must be contextualized in the transformation of the Far Right after the financial crisis of the beginning of the millenium during what has been termed the Great Regression, which has seen challenges not only to social but also to civil rights. The elections of Donald Trump in the US and of Jair Bolsonaro in Brazil (together with Brexit) were the main steps in the strengthening of the Far Right, which combined with strongly retrograde, neo-conservative and ultra-nationalist turns within populist discourses.

Although their positions and behaviour have varied as the pandemic progressed, far-right actors have provided important organizational resources and political opportunities for the spread of conspiracy theories and anti-vaccination positions in many countries, often associating the Covid-19 virus with immigration, especially 'illegal' immigration, as well as with ethnic minorities. While they have been somewhat divided on the question of restrictive measures, including lockdowns, the wearing of face masks, the enforcement of social distancing and the banning of large gatherings (measures that some of them initially supported), far-right parties have often sponsored anti-lockdown and even anti-vax positions, adopting conspiracy visions (Stavrakakis and Katsambekis 2020; Wondreys and Mudde 2022). As has also been found in the dismissal of anthropogenic explanations for global warming, there is a strong correlation between right-wing populist attitudes and anti-scientific beliefs, with experts considered to be part of the elite or at least subordinated to it and its assumed interests. The right-wing populist narrative is characterized by mistrust in scientists, who are viewed as being part of 'a broadly understood "elite"—one which secures the dominant ideas of an era—comprised of intellectuals, experts, scientists, institutions and cultural elites' (Galanopoulos and Venizelos 2022: 3).

In the anti-vax protests we will, in fact, see the convergence of specific developments on the Far Right that have accompanied the spread of backlash politics, defined as a period in which far-right politics has entered public discourse (Alter and Zürn 2020: 4) In short, we can consider backlash politics as characterized by the convergence of intensified organizational networking, increased capacity for collective actions and aggressive framing by retrograde actors (including movements) (della Porta 2020). This increase went hand in hand with a number of transformations that, as we shall see, influenced the development of the anti-vax protests. Research on the Far Right has often singled out anti-modernist frames, linked to exclusivist, nationalist, xenophobic, and anti-democratic positions (Eatwell 1996; Mudde 2007; Berezin 2009). Retrograde frames have often been used, with appeals to a supposed former purity of race. Following the increasing stigmatization of the discourse of ethnic superiority, old racist-supremacist frames have been blended into a new discourse of a defence of ethnic purity through separateness. In recent times, nativism has spread as 'an ideology which holds that states should be inhabited exclusively by members of the native groups (the nation) and that non-native elements (persons and ideas) are fundamentally threatening to the homogeneous nation-state' (Mudde 2007: 19). Similarly, anticapitalism is framed as a return to traditional values—albeit one that is accompanied by the promotion of national (and capitalist) economic interests and corporatist anti-class discourses. Within this populist turn, political and economic elites are seen as traitors to the nation and the economy. We will see how these trends are reflected in the focus on exclusive nationalism in the anti-vax protests, with a convergence in the New Age milieu on anti-EU and populist frames.

Moreover, traditional elements in the Far Right have been bridged with certain neo-conservative concerns, within what has been defined as a backlash against the moral revolution of progressive social movements in terms of women's rights, gender rights, and civil rights in general. In the 1990s, extreme right-wing politics was defined as an anti-modern and counter-revolutionary reaction against post-materialism (Perrineau 1997). In recent years, although selectively and unequally, a 'religious revival' has given new emphasis to the defence of traditional family values, which had already previously characterized the rhetoric of many fascist regimes and neofascist parties and movements. As recent research has singled out, the anti-gender movement, which claims to defend freedom of speech, thought and conscience, has politicized religious actors and discourse, allying with far-right actors. It has targeted in particular women's and LGBT rights, focusing on sexual and reproductive rights, same-sex marriage, adoption by same-sex parents, sexual education, the protection of women and gender minorities from violence, new reproductive technologies, as well as what they consider to be sexual permissiveness (Paternotte and Kuhar 2018). In the alliance with the Far Right, old frames have been bridged with new, emerging concerns.[7]

In several European countries the 2010s saw a transformation in the pro-life campaign, with the split of an anti-gender component. The pro-life mobilization had emerged in particular within the Catholic Church in support of the traditional family in the face of perceived challenges that go back to the UN International Conference on Population and Development in Cairo in 1994 and the UN Fourth World Conference on Women in Beijing in 1995. Considering the Church as far too oriented towards compromise on what was considered to be an anthropological challenge against the 'natural moral order', various groupings started to attack what they claimed was the strongest threat to the 'natural family', which was seen in the development of a discourse on gender and on gender rights, including the rights not only of women but also those of LGBTQ individuals. Developed within religious institutions and promoted by right-wing movement organizations and parties, anti-gender ideas have been bridged with the defence of traditional values and identities. In this discursive strategy, the rhetorical toolkit also includes the spreading of fear against minority groups, who are portrayed as perpetrators of attacks against the nation (ibid.). Calls for the protection of children resonated with the traditional opposition to state intervention in education and the proclamation of the freedom of parents in this domain. From an organizational point of view, the anti-gender campaigns were characterized by a loose coordination of a number of groupings, some of which amounted to no more than a logo, albeit with generous financing and a certain level of rootedness within religious structures and institutions. Inspired by the French *Manif pour Tous*, various groupings promoted street protests and allied with the Far Right, who offered them political channels. Empirical evidence will be presented in this volume that indicates a convergence

---

[7] Ambivalent positions have in fact pushed for a differentiation of far-right actors based on some crucial ideological features and the characteristics of the main groups that are targeted for exclusion in their discourse (Castelli Gattinara and Pirro 2018), within a shared rejection of diversity and aspiration to national homogeneity (Froio 2018; Mudde 2007; Taggart 2000; Minkenberg 2011).

within the anti-vax protests of an ultra-conservative milieu that appeals to the support of 'natural laws' against state intervention.

Within this development, ultraconservative claims have been connected with a defence of Western values. Resonating with a range of issues at the heart of right-wing authoritarian nativist ideology, the debate on the Charlie Hebdo attacks represented a further opportunity for far-right organizations to access the public sphere with the aim of exploiting fears, but also presenting themselves as champions of the Western civilization. In backlash politics, anti-Islamic rhetoric is at times framed as defense of freedom and tolerance (on the Charlie Hebdo debate, see della Porta et al. 2020). Thus, 'Far right organizations gained visibility in the public sphere by taking advantage of the resonance of liberal values in the wake of the Paris attacks, and actively mobilized to target cultural relativism and political correctness in their respective countries and at the European level' (ibid.: 121.).

At the same time, the anti-vax protest found space in the growing mistrust towards scientific knowledge. In particular, the cult of one's own body, and the aspiration for total freedom have been singled out as developmental trends in so-called New Age milieus (Speit 2021), especially in relation to its commercial turn and increasing individualism. The term New Age has been used to describe a heterogeneous set of spiritual, or even religious, practices that have developed in Western countries since the early 1970s. It has been presented as 'a common denominator for a variety of quite divergent contemporary popular practices and beliefs' (Hammer 2006: 855), including various groups and ideas converging in the 'expectation of a major and universal change being primarily founded on the individual and collective development of human potential' (York 1995: 2). With particular focus on 'everyday spirituality' (MacKian 2012: 12) and a core concern with healing practices, the New Age milieu has been said to mix theosophy and anthroposophy with the hippie counterculture of the 1960s and apocalyptic beliefs.

New Age activists often criticize rationalism and scientific methods, with some believing in individual karma and reincarnation. Disenchantment with mainstream society has brought about a focus on changing oneself instead of society as a whole. Self-spirituality has been linked to 'unmediated individualism', i.e., the belief that individual experience is the main source of authority on spiritual matters (Heelas 1996: 21). The calls for freedom and the autonomy of the individual, oriented towards personal growth, are grounded in a belief in the existence of a true Self (Hammer 2001) connected to a sort of divine essence of the universe (Hanegraaff 1996). This has been associated with both capitalism and late modernity, fuelling a belief in a free market of spiritual ideas as a parallel to the free market in economics (York 2001).

Locating Western civilization at the centre of a sequence of different 'ages' (Hanegraaff 1996), the New Age approach has been found to be especially widespread among white, highly educated middle- and upper-middle-class individuals, often women from the baby boomer generation, with a high presence of professional, managerial, artistic, and entrepreneurial occupations (Brown 1992; Heelas 1996; Sutcliffe 2003; Heelas and Woodhead 2005). However, degrees of commitment varied greatly between the converted and the consumers. In fact, it was noted that the majority of New Agers mainly participate through the purchase of books and products targeted at the New Age market, positioning the New Age movement as one that is primarily consumerist and commercial (Aldred 2000).

Looking at the milieu of alternative health practices, which has been associated with the environmental movement and progressive politics, research has pointed to its growing commercialization, with the development of narcissistic trends and strongly individualistic values (Kleffner and Meisner 2021). Indeed, calls for spirituality were associated with the growth of business activities around books, magazines, jewellery, and music (Sutcliffe 2003). The strong focus on alternative medicine and healing practices has been reflected in the creation of several enterprises that follow the assumption that in order to heal an illness one has to develop holistic practices that address the physical as well as the spiritual elements by stimulating so-called self-healing (Heelas 1996; MacKian 2012). This holistic view implies an assumption of connections between the body and the soul as well as between the individual and the universe, with the adoption of alternative practices ranging from acupuncture to chiropractic, yoga, aroma-, crystal-, or chromo-therapy, meditation and, especially, homeopathy as well as the establishment of separate schools for the education of children. Some New Age practitioners have even sponsored the use of spiritual techniques as a tool for attaining financial prosperity (Heelas 1996), with the development of specific New Age programmes for business people. This emphasis on commercial products has led to the interpretation of New Age beliefs as an expression of consumerism (Heelas 2006), narcissist tendencies and even the promotion of elitism, with New Age products becoming status symbols. The trust in alternative medicine has often been combined with anti-scientific trends, in particular against allopathic medicine, with a strong commercialization around homeopathic products, special diets, and so-called natural products. A schooling system inspired by anthroposophy and biodynamic agricultural practices has spread in parallel with these developments, in which greater value is given to personal achievements.

In at least part of this milieu, an extreme version of libertarianism has been bridged with a rejection of state interference in individual freedoms. A call for a return to nature and tradition has gone together with the narcissistic tendency aimed at the strengthening of one's own body and soul. These trends have been particularly visible in the debate around anthroposophical thinking. Moreover, regressive positions have been singled out in parts of the elitist Waldorf-schools and other initiatives promoted by the spiritualist movement inspired by Rudolf Steiner, who himself had been criticized for holding racist positions as well as for the authoritarian habitus of his spiritual vision, which were shared by some of his supporters that aligned on the Far Right (Speit 2021; Benz 2021a). While political positions have been fairly heterogeneous, some of the New Age producers commercializing non-Western practices have been accused of cultural imperialism (Heelas 2006).

Before the pandemic, conspiracies were already present in the New Age milieu in the form of the abovementioned alleged plot to steel personal data (including DNA information) through 5G technology, or to control people (or even kill them in order to reduce overpopulation) through 'chemical trails' spread by aeroplanes. Immediately prior to the pandemic, researchers had also begun to note the penetration in the New Age milieu of the politicized QAnon conspiracy which had been promoted by the Far Right. In Italy, a social scientist working on this milieu expressed her surprise when she noted the diffusion of QAnon conspiracy statements in the groups that she was observing:

If I had not known them so well, I would not have been so struck and unsettled by a widespread trend that, I suspect, the COVID-19 lockdown amplified and that my Facebook page recorded with zeal: their apparent 'belief' in conspiracy theories and, in particular, in the ones coming from overseas. Every day, for weeks up to the present moment, I have been witnessing many of my Pagan friends and acquaintances sharing, commenting, and posting many articles, YouTube videos, interviews, podcasts, and memes that portray a number of conspiracies. Some of them are related to the virus, some are animated by anti-vax stances, some are against the introduction of the 5G technologies. Some are conspiracy theories based in Italy; others are broadly international. Among the conspiracies that circulate in these Pagan networks of belonging are claims that COVID-19 is the result of genetic engineering and escaped from a lab; Coronavirus is not more lethal than a 'simple' flu; the declaration of pandemic (and not, 'merely', of epidemic) was done in the attempt of get us all vaccinated or to install a microchip under our skin so that we can be controlled; COVID-19 was created to financially speculate on the vaccine; and COVID-19 is created or accelerated by 5G technology. Moreover, in the spring of 2020, two videos went viral among my interlocutors and have been extremely influential: Plandemic, featuring Dr. Judy Mikovits, and an interview with Dr. Shiva Ayyadurai by The Next News Network. As a matter of fact, and to my surprise, some of the conspiracies that circulate among my interlocutors include North American ones on the 'deep state', linked to QAnon, and anti-vax theories fostered by Robert F. Kennedy Jr.

(ibid.: 508)

It is not by chance that encounters had already taken place between the Far Right and the New Age milieu prior to the pandemic. A particularly notable point of networking were the previous campaigns against the compulsory vaccination of children or vaccination campaigns for elderly people, in which anti-vax New Age milieus had met with ultra-conservative religious groups that are hostile to any form of state regulation in the name of the Church's prerogative. In this manner anti-gender frames were connected with calls for home schooling, against the public lay school system, and in favour of the sole responsibility of parents for their children's medical treatment. The spread of conspiracy beliefs in the New Age milieu has also been a general trend; indeed, this has led to the coining of the term 'conspirituality', conceptualized as 'the relationships between New Age spirituality and conspiracy theories' (Parmigiani 2021: 506).

In particular, anti-vax protests have been seen as confirming a normalization (Wodak 2019) of the Far Right, due to the fact that other actors participating in the protests generally seemed happy to express solidarity with their neo-fascist allies. As has been observed in the case of the German anti-vax protests, 'The organisers and those actively participating seem not to care about the presence and co-option by the Far Right; this is a repercussion of the normalisation of far-right views: Whereas these protest movements cannot be labelled far-right populist, their anti-elite anger and willingness to share platforms with neo-Nazis, anti-Semites, and *Reichsburger*, confirms the argument for the normalisation of far-right orientations' (Vieten 2020: 11).

As we shall see, the analysis of the anti-vax protests will point to the relevance of the specific evolution of the various waves that often compose cycles, considering the transformation in the forms of action and the involved actors following mechanisms of imitation and competition. My research on the anti-vax protests will point to the further convergence of a variety of different nets that had already been in contact during previous campaigns against other vaccination campaigns, but also against gender rights. The Far Right played an important role in resource mobilization by instrumentally broadening their appeals in order to attract support from within a commercialized New Age milieu as well as an ultra-conservative anti-gender milieu that provided an individualist and anti-state narrative as well as a blend of conspiratorial visions.

Analysing the anti-vax protests

In this volume, I will address anti-vax protests through a processual approach that is both context- and time-sensitive, taking into consideration the complex relational, affective, and cognitive dynamics at play during the evolution of contentious politics.

Social movement studies have focused attention on the dynamics that move from structure into action. The role of grievances as precipitating factors or turning points is, in fact, mediated by existing social movement organizations (Staggenborg 1993) and, more generally, movement networks that mobilize collective resources. The research presented in this volume focuses on the sets of questions that are related to how pandemic grievances fuelled protests against anti-contagion measures thanks to the activation of specific social movement families. As mentioned above, while concerns with inequalities were represented by progressive movements with claims for social justice, the rejection of anti-contagion measures (up to the refusal of vaccination) was instead promoted by retrograde movements, with claims for unconstrained individual freedom. In order to understand the dynamics of mobilization on the retrograde side, the analysis presented here develops around three main concepts in the literature on social movement studies: repertoires of contention, organizational networks and collective frames (della Porta and Diani 2020). I consider these movement characteristics to be influenced by contextual opportunities as well as specific organizational resources, evolving within broad relational fields of interaction during the course of the mobilization.

With regard to the first of these, social movement studies have paid particular attention to *protest*, as one of the main expressions of emerging grievances. Cycles of protest, in particular, have been connected with the opening up of certain opportunities for the expression of societal conflicts. The specific repertoires of contention have been seen to vary in time and space, adapting to changing circumstances. At the same time, however, they tend to be constrained by the traditions of the specific social movements and social movement organizations that employ them, being adapted to the amount and type of resources available for them as well as constrained by their specific normative choices. In the course of their development during protest cycles,

forms of action might change, with both radicalization and institutional-
ization representing potential paths. The empirical analysis of *protest waves*
against the anti-contagion measures during the Covid-19 pandemic will
point to the symbolic radicalization of the protest forms, with a convergence
of the Far Right with the New Age milieu.

Secondly, social movement studies have generally linked *organizational*
choices to both material resources and normative preferences. Social movements typically do not identify with one single organization, but are instead
made up of networks of different individuals and groups who are often
also active in arenas other than protest. While certainly influenced by their
environment, social movement organizations are guided not solely by strategic considerations, but also by normative concerns. The selection of an
organizational model does not only follow rational assessments concerning the allocation of tasks, but is also constrained by existing organizational
repertoires and assessments of appropriateness with quite different organizational models being employed by progressive and regressive movements. The
research presented in this volume develops an analysis of the specific organizational structure of the anti-vax movement, based on a collective action
mode which I conceptualize as a *disembedded crowdsourced* model, in which
movement entrepreneurs distribute resources for mobilization that are aimed
at specific constituencies who are invited to self-organize. While this model
resonates with the liquid context in which protest develops, it also proves
weak in promoting resilience when mobilization declines, given its weak level
of embeddedness in broad movement networks.

Thirdly, social movement studies points to *frames* as defining the dominant world views that guide the behaviour of social movement organizations
and activists. Framing processes have been considered to be the instrumental
dimension of the symbolic construction of reality by collective entrepreneurs
and are very often strategically produced by the organizational leadership. In
order for a grievance to emerge, a specific strain must be linked in a logical
manner to criticism of the ways in which authorities treat social problems.
While grievances originate in material conditions, triggering feelings of dissatisfaction, resentment, or indignation, the decision to mobilize on those
grievances requires cognitive processes. In general, the responsibility for the
unpleasant situation needs to be attributed to a deliberate producer. In times
of crisis, framing is all the more relevant given the high levels of uncertainty and therefore the need to find explanations for unknown situations.
In order to convince individuals to act, frames must point at the relevance
of a given problem to individual life experiences. Along with the critique
of dominant representations of order and of social patterns, frames must

therefore produce new definitions of the foundations of collective identification. Within this tradition, I will analyse the diagnostic and prognostic framing by anti-vax actors, thus distinguishing a definition of the self, often linked to motivational frames, and a definition of the opponents, i.e., the 'others' against which the mobilization is oriented. I will suggest that *conspiracy beliefs* helped to connect the Far Right with anti-gender groupings and a New Age milieu, which brought about a focus on individual freedom and personal responsibility as embedded in alternative health practices.

The analysis of the evolution of the anti-vax mobilization will point at the presence of sectarian dynamics. In general, ideology plays a particularly important integrative function the more a group is subject to strong centrifugal pressures, given fragmentation and isolation, becoming 'one of the main tools which can be used to guarantee integration' (Melucci 1990: 6). Accordingly, movement ideologies exalt powerful, strong, and abstract ideas, as the transcendence of factual arguments makes ideological beliefs more resistant to external defeats. Bringing this to the extreme, political sects tend to idealize the value of living outside normal standards, the idea of courage as a duty of the true believer, and the commitment to sacrifice as shared suffering (Kanter 1968, 1972). Dogmatic ideologies, offering a high degree of certainty about the external world, help to motivate radical behaviour (Gerlach and Hine 1970). The actual content of ideologies that are characteristic of small radical organizations favours the ideal of a closed community of the elect, emphasizing purity rather than proselytization, exclusivity rather than expansion (O'Toole 1977). Elitism makes isolation appear a positive, self-imposed condition. The inner versus outer mentality thus fuels a dichotomous image of the world (Gerlach and Hine 1970). As Lofland (1985: 224) observed, some groups 'tend to look out over the social landscape with suspicion, fear and hostility, and quantitatively to restrict their contact with people unlike themselves, most particularly with people who are only in small ways unlike themselves'. Research on specific forms of collective action, such as clandestine political organizations or civil wars, has shown how sectarian dynamics can emerge out of isolation, affecting the micro-mobilization processes, but also the organizational models and eventually the general societal context (della Porta 1995, 2013). Several of these dynamics seem to apply to the evolution of the anti-vax actors during the Covid-19 pandemic. As will be argued in what follows, conspiracy theories can be considered as playing a similar integration role in the anti-vax protests, strengthening internal integration, while at the same time increasing external stigmatization. A conspiracy mindset can, therefore, spread through a vicious cycle, as a reaction to (actual and perceived) isolation that strengthens said isolation.

By comparing the evolution of the anti-vax protest in different countries, this research aims to assess how processual dynamics and contextual constraints and opportunities interacted in both time and space. In this direction, I will look at how political conditions influenced the alliance structure of anti-vax protestors, but also at how preceding mobilizing structures impacted on the repertoires of action, organizational models and collective framing of the anti-vax protests. From a processual perspective, I will also consider how the dynamics of contentious politics evolved during various moments of the pandemic.

The research and this volume

The empirical research begins by addressing the Italian context, which I consider as a crucial case study for the analysis of contentious politics during the pandemic. It then expands the discussion from a comparative perspective, by presenting empirical research as well as secondary analysis of existing studies on further two cases, Germany and Greece, considered to be paradigmatic of different types of anti-vax mobilization. Following this, secondary analysis will be presented from other countries in Europe and North America with the aim of discussing the generalizability of the evidence collected.

Italy is considered a critical case study given that it was the first country after China to be hit by the spread of the Covid-19 virus, with the most dramatic consequences in the first wave of the pandemic between February and May 2020. While in the medium term it was eventually overtaken by other countries in terms of the rate of Covid-19 cases in the population, given the particular lethality of the virus in the spring of 2020, Italy remained imprinted on the global collective memory as the country that had to deal with the health catastrophe in its most acute phase and when less information was available on the virus and as a result on how to cure infected individuals. The images of army trucks transporting the bodies of the many of victims that could not be buried in the cemetery of Bergamo provoked a deep emotional impact well beyond the country.

As the country in which the virus initially arrived in Europe, with northern regions suffering an incredibly quick spread of the pandemic and a particularly lethal impact, Italy also represents a highly relevant case due to the early development of institutional responses aimed at curbing the contagion, which were both very severe and long-lasting. Indeed, after Wuhan in China, the first severe lockdown measures were enacted in Italy, including shelter-in-place orders in the very first months of the pandemic. Moreover, in the successive stages of the outbreak, Italy was among the first countries to implement curfews as well as the use of vaccination certificates, up to and including compulsory vaccination for members of certain professions and senior citizens. Although the initial shock at the scale of the virus led to a high degree of support for government orders to shelter in place, over time critical reactions also developed against the very rigorous anti-contagion measures put in place, especially after the perception of the danger of the virus had started to subside. In spite of the fact that they only involved a very small section of the population, the anti-vax protests were able to attract a great deal of attention over a relatively extended period of time.

As of October 2022, Covid-19 had led to 179,000 deaths in Italy, and 23.5 million people were officially counted as having been infected by the virus. The most dramatic peak was during the first wave. The excess mortality rate in 2020 compared to the average of the previous five years, was 100,526 deaths— the highest number since the end of WWII. Covid-19 officially arrived in January 2020, spreading quickly throughout the country, with the first deaths taking place as early as February, when eleven municipalities in Northern Italy were put under lockdown. This measure was then expanded to the entire country on 11 March, when all commercial activities (with the sole exception of pharmacies and large food chains) as well as non-essential business were closed down and citizens' movements drastically reduced, a situation that remained in place until 3 June. In October 2020, the emergence of a second wave of Covid-19 was addressed with the introduction of a new lockdown. The lockdown, including curfews, was once again lifted in June 2021; however, with cases increasing again, the government introduced the Green Pass (certifying vaccination, recovery from Covid-19 infection or a negative test result) which it made compulsory for accessing many sites and activities. At a later stage, the key requirements became proof of vaccination or recovery. Italy also implemented compulsory vaccination in the health, education, and police sectors and in January 2022 mandated vaccination for all citizens above the age of 50 (even if the only penalty for violation of the obligation was a €100 fine). By October 2022, 80% of the entire population had been vaccinated.

Germany, with its 154,000 deaths and 35.7 million infected citizens up to October 2022, is another country that has certainly suffered a great deal during the pandemic. While it had largely succeeded in containing the first wave through the very early measures of lockdown (including the closure of educational institutions as well as curfews) and the closing of borders, in the autumn of 2020 the second wave hit hard, notwithstanding the harsher lockdown measures introduced in December 2020 and January 2021. While many measures varied by member state, faced with a third wave in the spring of

2021, the Infection Protection Act increased the powers of the federal government to impose anti-contagion measures. However, the strictest policies only came into place in the summer of 2021, when the fourth wave triggered the adoption of so called 3G rules that made being either vaccinated, recovered or tested a condition to access various venues. With daily infection levels rising to several tens of thousands per day, the strengthened 3G+ rules imposed vaccination as a condition for accessing shops and other recreational places as well as public transport, although it did fall short of making vaccination compulsory for at least some professions. Notwithstanding the efforts of the new Public Health Minister in the SPD-Green-FDP government, Karl Lauterbach, vaccination rates remained relatively low, with 76% of citizens fully vaccinated in the autumn of 2022 and a high degree of difference between states (with extremely low values in eastern states in particular).

Greece, with 33,750 deaths and 5.2 million people infected up to October 2022, was one of the European countries that, although managing to keep the first wave under control, saw high levels of contagion later on. In March 2020, while levels of infection were very low (and with seventeen deaths), the Greek government imposed a lockdown, which was then lifted in the summer and re-established in November after a surge of infections in the second wave of contageon. This was once again introduced in reaction to the third wave in the Winter of 2021, including restrictions on movement and gatherings as well as travel and entry restrictions. With a very vulnerable public health system, given the cuts imposed during the financial crisis, anti-contagion measures tended to be particularly strict, especially outside of the tourist season, with high police visibility in the repression of violation of anti-contagion measures. As in the German and the Italian cases, from the summer of 2021 onwards these anti-contagion measures included the widespread use of vaccination certificates to access public places and, as in the Italian case but in contrast with Germany, compulsory vaccination for workers in the educational, health and police sectors as well as for the elderly. In October 2022, 71% of the population were fully vaccinated with the centre-right government refusing to invest public funds in order to structurally strengthen the public health system.

As for the empirical analysis, in studying the Italian case, I will rely on original empirical research on the anti-vax protests related to the Covid-19 pandemic in Italy in the period 2020–1. The research is based on a protest event analysis covering the years 2020 and 2021, an organizational analysis based on organizational documents collected online and a frame analysis based on publications in various channels of communication. In addition to this, the results of ongoing academic research projects as well as reports produced by non-governmental organizations, institutions and print media were taken into account.

One of the main empirical sources for my study is protest event analysis, which is a quantitative methodology that is widely used to study the dynamics of contentious politics in time and space. As synthesized by Koopmans and Rucht, protest event analysis 'is a method that allows for the quantification of many properties of protest, such as frequency, timing and duration, location, claims, size, forms, carriers, and targets, as well as immediate consequences and reactions (e.g., police intervention, damage, counter protests)' (2002: 231). In general, daily press reports represent the source for this analysis, where articles on protest are found and coded following specific methods of content analysis (Kriesi et al. 1995; Hutter 2014; Lindekilde 2014). In this process, the primary unit of analysis is the protest event, and information is collected on indicators that usually include the actors who are involved in the event, the forms of action they use, their claims, and their targets, as well as the place, time, and immediate outcomes of the protest.

While extremely helpful in defining broad trends in collective action, protest event analysis must be handled with care (Hutter 2014) as the reporting of protests is quite selective, and selectivity is often a source of bias given the fact that the portion of the universe of protest events that is reported is never a representative (or a random) sample but rather—pour cause— influenced by the logic of the media. In this sense, not only do events that mobilize large number of protestors, use more innovative forms, or escalate into violence have a higher chance of being reported, but the claims on which people mobilized can be considered more or less newsworthy (McCarthy, McPhail, and Smith 1996; Fillieule and Jiménez 2003; Hutter 2014). Reporting can also be more or less detailed and neutral according to the characteristics of the actors and forms of actions. Additionally, the more frequent a protest becomes, the more selective reporting on it will be. While acknowledging these biases, researchers have noted that since protest is an act of communication, protest event analysis captures those events that have already passed an initial important threshold in influencing public opinion and policymakers: being reported upon (Rucht and Ohlemacher 1992). Moreover, as with any source, it is essential to be self-reflexive in the interpretation of the data as well as triangulating newspaper-based protest event analysis with the reporting of protests in other sources.

For this research, protest event analysis has covered the period from 1 April 2020 to 31 March 2022. This timeframe starts with the onset of the first protests against the first lockdown—which officially began on 9 March 2020—and ends with the steep decline of protests in March 2022, making it possible to observe the evolution of the protest waves throughout an almost two-year period (della Porta and Lavizzari 2022). Following an established practice in protest event analysis (Hutter 2014), we systematically searched for events on the Italian daily 'La Repubblica' (national pages) using the search string '(Protest* OR manifest*) AND (lockdown OR no vax* OR vaccin* OR chiusur* OR Green pass*)'. La Repubblica has been selected (as has often been the case in earlier research based on protest event analysis in Italy) as it has an extensive and deep coverage of protest events, given that the national pages tend to report the news also present in the different local editions of the same newspaper (i.e., Rome, Milan, Bari, Bologna, Florence, Genoa, Naples, Palermo, Parma, and Turin). The search through a list of keyword strings is consistent with previous research using protest event analysis (ibid.); the specific strings used were chosen in order to retrieve a wide variety of protest forms and events involving the topics of vaccination, lockdown and containment measures, closures of activities, as well as the vaccination certificate (Green Pass). A sample search on selected local editions (Rome, Milan, Genoa, Naples, Turin) revealed no additional cases to those already included in the database of events reported in the national edition. The pertinent articles were then selected and all events found were coded (N = 114) using a codebook. Specifically, information has been coded on the date and place of the events, the forms of action, the organizers, number of participants, the claims, and the target.

In order to control for the selection bias of the protest event analysis, we also consulted some of the websites and social media pages of the main protest coordinator bodies (such as Fronte del Dissenso, or the Dissent Front). In addition to the protest event analysis conducted through quantitative techniques, the data was also triangulated through a qualitative analysis of other newspaper articles and news feeds with open search by forms of action, which made it possible to enrich the description of the protest events, most notably when reporting information on the repertoires of action. In addition to this, video content analysis was also performed. As research on social movement communication has often noted, social movement activists are (increasingly) using cameras to record protest events as well as posting their videos on social media and various other platforms. In addition, journalists also tend to use visuals to a greater extent in their coverage of protests, publishing videos on contentious events on the websites of newspapers. In this context, video analysis can greatly contribute to both ethnographic approaches (by allowing for a broadening of the events covered and a reduction of costs) as well as protest event analysis, making it possible to integrate the written coverage by journalists, which is often very short and, naturally, largely mediated by the journalists' consideration of the newsworthiness of the topic, as well as the information available to the journalists themselves (della Porta et al. forthcoming).

The video content analysis of four major protest events covering different periods supplements a qualitative dimension to our analysis. The videos were sampled based on their availability online and the saliency of the events recorded, covering the period of autumn 2020, spring 2021, and two events in autumn 2021, allowing us to extend the analysis over the two main waves. The videos were uploaded by the protest organizers themselves, on their social media pages, or by reporters through the 'Local Team' platform, a public and free online video platform for live images of different types of events taking place in Italy. In total, twenty-five videos were sampled and analysed, varying in length from two minutes to two hours. For the video analysis, a specific 'Observation template for virtual ethnography and content analysis' was created (della Porta et al. forthcoming). The data thus collected on banners, slogans, chants, and speeches provide information on the self-representation of the protestors as well as the diagnostic and prognostic frames relating to the pandemic. Video analysis also made it possible to obtain some information on the participants in the events as well as on the general atmosphere, while also allowing to collect data resembling more 'classical' content analysis.

The protest event analysis allowed us to single out some of the main organizations for the study of organizational models and collective framing employed. The empirical analysis of the organizational structure of anti-vax protestors in Italy is based then on documents produced by the anti-vax groups themselves, especially those uploaded to the websites, Facebook accounts, and blogs of the groups in question. The selection of the groups covered in the research was initially based on the abovementioned protest event analysis of anti-vax mobilizations, which made it possible to single out a list of organizations that were mentioned as promoters of the protest. The sample was then expanded through snowballing, thus including different types of organizations that were found to be connected with the first set of groups. Expert interviews were conducted in order to complete the case selections. The analysis, conducted on organizational statutes and relevant documents, addressed the organizational format, including degrees of formalization, internal decision-making, conceptions of membership, and leadership.

The frame analysis covered texts published on the internet by the main groupings and organizations involved in the protests against measures such as lockdowns, face masks, social distancing, the Green Pass, and the vaccination campaign. Initially, information was collected on the umbrella groups that called for protest events on these issues, subsequently snowballing on their organizational contacts online and the documents that they shared. The main focus was on websites and Facebook accounts, while blogs were also examined. From these sources, a range of data were downloaded, including documents related to Covid-19 as well as the 'who we are' section and, when available, the organizational statutes. This material was then analysed through iterative reading. First, the material was read through, and the main content was singled out. Keywords were then listed and subsequently organized around diagnostic, prognostic, identity, and oppositional statements, aggregating the content around a number of subsets within the respective frames.

This research was replicated, as much as was possible, in the German and Greek case studies, which are considered as highly relevant for a cross-national comparison, as the former is the European country in which anti-vax protests first became visible and then remained sustained for the longest period, while the latter is taken as an illustration of the low mobilizing capacity of the anti-vax movement. For both cases, the research was expanded through a secondary analysis of existing research.

Building on social movement studies, this work looks at how the anti-vax protests developed. The three chapters that follow this introduction will each deal with one of three main concepts used for the analysis of contentious politics, which will be introduced and discussed in each of them in turn: namely the repertoires of contention, resource mobilization and collective framing. Chapter 2 looks at the repertoires of contention, analysing the main forms of collective action used in two different waves of protest, with particular attention paid to processes of *radicalization*. Chapter 3 analyses the organizational structures of the protests, identifying a *disembedded crowdsourced* model based on the online provision of toolkits designed for self-mobilization. Chapter 4 addresses the collective framing of the protests, assessing how *conspiracy* theories supported the definition of the diagnosis and of the prognosis, with the convergence of various groups around the narrative of a 'global Reset' with the nonvaccinated presented as victims of a 'sanitary dictatorship', but also as the saviours of humanity. The conclusion reflects on resource mobilization within the movement networks as well as on the contextual opportunities and constraints for anti-vax protests.

2

Anti-vax Protests

Singling Out Waves within Cycles

The repertoire of action: Radicalization processes

In Italy, the period of the first lockdown saw only very sporadic, small symbolic action against the anti-contagion measures. With the pandemic killing thousands, strict measures of isolation were generally welcomed and protests rather called for more health security measures for those who could not stay at home. When, in June 2020, the shelter-in-place orders were lifted (even if other measures, such as facial masks but also restrictions in movement, were still in place), hope emerged that the pandemic would end in the Summer and not come back. If not yet a new pandemic wave, the Summer however brought with it dare economic conditions, especially for the workers—particularly those under precarious work contracts—and small entrepreneurs in the tourist and the catering sector. With a resurgence of contagion and casualties related with Covid-19 virus in the early Fall, and further anti-contagion measures announced, some protest events were called, targeting especially the new lock-down and related curfew. Some escalation, with street fight with the police, happened in Florence on 30 October. The protest was called through an unsigned leaflet, spread on the social media and on WhatsApp, that invited citizens to meet in Piazza della Signoria and 'flex their muscles' against the anti-Covid measures. The main slogan in the short leaflet was 'Let's circulate Florence' ('Fate girare Firenze')—a statement which played with the overlapping meanings of forwarding the news, circulating against the lockdown and let Florence be dynamic again. The public authorities as well as the media stigmatized the call for protest as irresponsible given the threat the virus still posed, while at the same time recognizing the legitimacy of the economic claims by some sectors of the population. Fear of violent escalation were mentioned, with accusation against those who wanted to 'manipulate the outrage' (so the

Regressive Movements in Times of Emergency. Donatella della Porta, Oxford University Press. © Donatella della Porta (2023).
DOI: 10.1093/oso/9780198884309.003.0002

Florentine mayor Nardella); the promoters of the protests remained anonymous. Videos published on line show very young people, moving in small groups, in part masked (also beyond the required facial mask), and with quite aggressive postures. Protestors (mostly using facial masks) were in fact filmed while damaging planters, dustbins and traffic posts as well as throwing stones and bottles at the police, in anti-riots equipment, that charged three times in the city center. Some protestors used smoke bombs, but also Molotov cocktails; the police responded with teargas. The only visible symbol were Italian flags, with the word 'Ora Basta' (enough now) written on one of them. A hand-made poster criticised the cut in the public health system, calling for 'free covid-tests for all'; another small one, carried by two women, called for 'hugs instead of masks". In a group of protesters showing more aggressive postures, one of them was filmed while addressing a small group of a dozen people, lamenting forced inactivity and hinting at related economic consequences: "we are police slaves, we cannot move, we cannot even walk around. We have to stay at home and wait for a subsidy". In a small group of protestors who did not take part in violence, participants stated: "Florence is dead", and asked "Where is the money promised by the government? Among the dozens of protestors arrested, 23 will be charged for damaging public and private property, resisting police arrests, non authorized protest and the making and using of inflammable objects. In the media and by the police, they are presented as young, professional trouble-makers from antagonist milieus, but also as coming from social category heavily hit by the pandemic crisis.

Based on an analysis of videos, this short account reports on one of the first visible protests against anticontageon measures. After the protest, whose violence was stigmatized by all political parties and association, a new lockdown entered in force, including however economic support for the activities that were penalized by it. No other violent protest related with anti-contagion measure was registered in Florence in the following years. Nevertheless, other forms of protests developed and radicalized, attacking anti-pandemic measures, among which vaccination. This chapter is devoted to the characteristics and evolution of these protests.

Within the field of social movement studies there has long been a particular focus on the question of contentious events, with a recognition of the fact that protests are not distributed randomly but instead tend to cluster in time and space through 'a punctuated history of heightened challenges and relative stability' (Beissinger 2002: 16). One of the first concepts introduced in order to describe this phenomenon is that of a protest cycle, defined as

> a phase of heightened conflict and contention across the social system that includes: a rapid diffusion of collective action from more mobilized to less mobilized sectors; a quickened pace of innovation in the forms of contention; new or transformed collective action frames; a combination of organised and unorganised participation; and sequences of intensified interactions between challengers and authorities which can end in reform, repression and sometimes revolution.
>
> **(Tarrow 1994: 153)**

During these cycles, protest rises and declines following a number of specific sequences, often moving 'from institutional conflict to enthusiastic peak to ultimate collapse' (ibid.: 168). However, other concepts such as tides or campaigns have also been introduced in order to refer to specific moments of intensification of collective action. As I will suggest in this chapter, cycles include specific waves, made up of protests focusing on similar claims within shorter periods of time. The interaction of various actors and mobilizations during such waves has an impact on the dynamics of a protest cycle, which have, in fact, been proven to vary over time and across space (della Porta, Gunzelmann, and Portos 2021).

Cycles are produced by the contentious mobilization of a large number and a wide range of actors, including various specific waves of protests focusing on similar aims. Mechanisms of imitation, competition and reciprocal learning regularly occur, triggering the intensification and de-intensification of protest waves. During the ascending phases of a cycle, precipitating circumstances produce a radical destabilization of social relations within a polity, and the increased unpredictability of interactions favours the diffusion of protest, as movements borrow (successful) inventions from each other (Koopmans 2004). By demonstrating the vulnerability of the authorities, the first movements to emerge lower the cost of collective action for other actors (Tarrow 1994). Through a process of imitation and learning, spin-off movements mobilize, sometimes in alliance with, sometimes in opposition to, the previous ones (della Porta and Tarrow 1986). As we shall see, however, actors and interactions change in different moments, making it possible to single out specific waves with their own ups and downs within the broader cycle.

Organizational dynamics are also involved in the development of the specific waves, with certain actors taking the lead in each of them. Social movement organizations cooperate and compete with each other, investing resources in order to intensify mobilization, winning or losing ground in different moments. Forms of action also tend to vary within each wave, with moments of radicalization and de-radicalization, new forms of action emerging as forms of protest which were once innovative tend to lose their newsworthiness, and state repression adapting and contributing to the transformation in the forms of action. The evolution of the cycle of contention varies, therefore, as it is influenced by the specific dynamics of the protest waves within it.

The anti-vax protests were part of a moment of intensification of contentious politics, which developed through the mobilization of various social and political actors that triggered different waves of contestation. In this chapter, I aim to zoom in on the cycle of protest that developed within the pandemic, singling out two different waves of contention targeting anti-contagion measures. An investigation of their evolution over time will make it possible to single out both the different composition and formats that characterized the various waves, as well as a number of elements of continuity between them. These would seem all the more relevant in assessing two of the main characteristics observed in earlier research on anti-vax protests, namely the heterogeneity of the actors and their radical potential.

With regard to the former, a typical image of the protests analysed here points to the diversity of the actors involved. Thus, for instance, in the United States, protests have been described as populated by 'anti-vaccination activists, gun rights advocates, adherents of the QAnon conspiracy theory, members of private armed militias, and Trump supporters' (Stavrakakis and Katsambekis 2020: 55). Similarly, in a number of European countries, anti-vax mobilizations have included a mix of the exoteric, New Age milieu and radical-right activists, with some promoters openly endorsing QAnon conspiracies and the far right providing important organizational resources.

Secondly, in initial research on the topic, the tactics of anti-vax protests have been shown to be characterized by confrontational strategies. It has been noted that:

the tactics adopted by protesters revolve around upsetting lockdown measures by the very fact of gathering in public space, without wearing protective equipment as a means of provocation. The flouting of mask-wearing and social distancing norms becomes in-and-of-itself a means through which non-compliance with government regulations and criticism at the management of the pandemic, and its economic consequences, can be aired.

(Gerbaudo 2020: 69)

The contentious repertoire included actions 'that disrupt or obstruct vaccination sites; attempts to sabotage vaccine doses; and reactionary legislative efforts prohibiting localities, schools and private businesses from enforcing mask usage guidelines, vaccine requirements, or policies to verify an individual's COVID-19 vaccination status' (Snow and Bernatzky 2023). Aggressive behaviour took on more radical forms, especially in countries such as the United States, with anti-vax 'demonstrators wielding semi-automatic rifles and other firearms, meant as symbols of popular sovereignty against the perceived oppression of government elites' (Stavrakakis and Katsambekis 2020: 65).

In order to assess both the variety and the radicality of the protests, in what follows, data from protest event analysis and video data analysis on the Italian case will be used to look first at the time and spatial evolution of the protests, then at the actors present in them, and finally the forms of action employed. In particular, I will demonstrate the diversity between the two waves of protests, which were in fact separated by a low ebb. Following this, I will compare the Italian case with the German and the Greek cases, looking at the former as an example of sustained protest and at the latter as one of very limited anti-vax contention. I will conclude with some general observations on the interaction of waves within cycles, which I believe is an important theoretical contribution to the protest event analysis.

The characteristics of the protests in time and space

The analysis of the protests in Italy between April 2020 and March 2022 singles out a marked diversity in the distribution and intensity of collective action in the broad period addressed. First of all, the number of protests *fluctuated*, with two major waves of contention separated by a period of low ebb (Figure 2.1a): the first wave extended from April to December 2020, and the second wave lasted from July to December 2021. Indeed, after the first lockdown in March and April 2020, the protests became more visible, initially as vigils, with marches subsequently organized in several cities throughout Italy. Initially small and localized, they occasionally grew in size as the first national protest events were organized, only to decline cyclically in parallel with the reduction in the rate of contagion.

The first wave of contestation is therefore characterized by protests against anti-contagion measures, such as the compulsory wearing of face masks, but especially against specific lockdown measures. In particular, protests first began to intensify in the autumn of 2020, with marches against the introduction of new lockdowns and curfews taking place at a local level, including some cases of escalation in fights between the protestors and the police, which however remained short and sporadic.

The second wave of contestation mostly centred on protests against the vaccination campaign and the vaccination certificate. After a long period of low mobilization between January and June 2021, when some of the previous claims had been met through the policy of state economic support for some economic sectors, protests escalated once again, especially against the decision taken by the government in the summer of 2021 to require a Green Pass (Covid vaccination certificate) and subsequently of selective compulsory vaccination to access public places and business. Not by chance, content related to the issue on Twitter peaked in July and November 2021, becoming fiercely polarized (Pilati and Micoli 2022).

Indeed, it was in the second half of 2021 that most of the protest events took place, with an increasing level of participation in the months of October to December (Figure 2.1b). The protests, which had already become intense in the summer of 2021, suddenly increased in intensity as the mandatory use of the vaccination certificate was progressively extended to more contexts, such as sports events, music festivals, bars and restaurants, gyms, and long-distance public transport. On 24 July 2021, coordinated protests were carried out in Naples, Turin, Milan, Genoa, and Rome, with the participation of

(a)

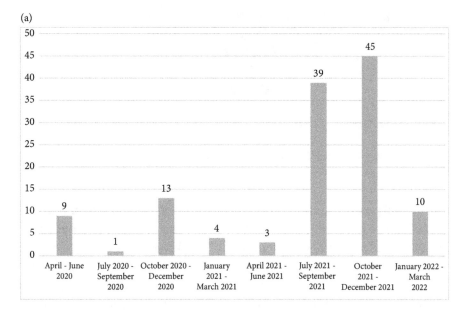

Figure 2.1a Number of protest events by quarter

(b)

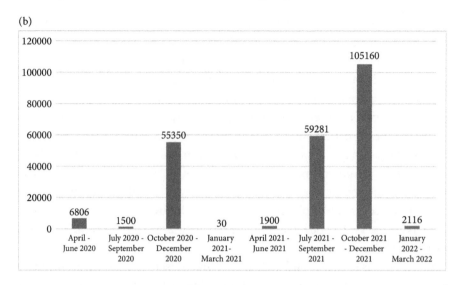

Figure 2.1b   Total number of participants by quarter

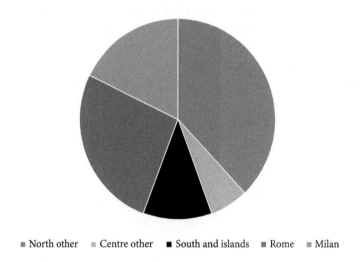

■ North other   ▦ Centre other   ■ South and islands   ■ Rome   ▦ Milan

Figure 2.2   Geographical distribution of the events

around 3000 people chanting 'Freedom', 'No Green Pass!', and 'Down with the dictatorship!'. Protest intensified further as, starting from 15 October 2021, the Green Pass mandate was extended to all workplaces.

In general, the protests were *mainly local and territorially concentrated*, with a few significant national events during the second wave. The majority of the protests took place in the North of Italy, with events concentrated in Milan, but also in the capital, Rome, in the centre of Italy (Figure 2.2).

The protest actors

Heterogeneity was also noted in relation to the main actors, as the *organizers of the protest events changed in terms of social and political groups*, with considerable differences in the two waves also noted here. Initially more spontaneous, they first involved the social groups most affected by the measures introduced to control the pandemic, with a subsequent shift to mainly ideological opponents of vaccination during the second wave. Politically, there was also an increasing influence of the Far Right in the organization of the protests, especially in cities such as Rome (see Figure 2.3).

In the first wave of protest, between April and December 2020, one can observe a mobilization of especially those social groups most heavily hit by the lockdown measures, with the loose coordination of small local events. The organizers of these protests, which most of the time were launched online through social media platforms (i.e., Telegram), were often little-known groupings, with no official webpages or communication sites.

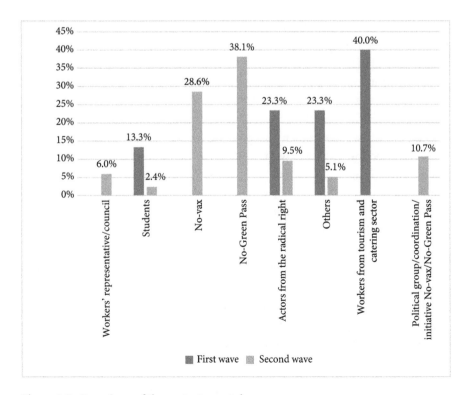

Figure 2.3 Organizers of the protest events by wave

As shown in Figure 2.3, the majority of the protest events during the first wave of contention were attended by a diverse set of social groups affected by the lockdown and anti-contagion measures, such as workers in the tourism and catering sector, students calling for the reopening of schools, as well as artists, high-school teachers, taxi drivers, and club owners (included in the 'Others' category in Figure 2.3). At times they were joined by people belonging to the economic and work sectors that had been most affected by the lockdown (notably in the restaurant, entertainment and tourism sectors), but also by football ultras and (more rarely) by squatted social centres. However, these protests were not supported by the business associations of shop owners, which instead employed other forms of collective actions.

The localized mode also continued to characterize the protests in the second wave in the summer and autumn of 2021; however, this period also saw a change in the type of groups promoting the protests and specific coordination groups were formed in various cities (e.g., *Variante Torinese* for Turin or *Libera Piazza Genova*[1]). In the second half of 2021 especially, some attempts were made at building national groups, which were often in competition with each other. One such group was *Basta Dittatura* ('End the Dictatorship'), which was founded in July 2021 to coordinate protests. The group created and distributed visual material online, including slogans or posters, such as photos of the then Prime Minister Mario Draghi depicted as Hitler. Moreover, according to some reports, *Basta Dittatura* gave instructions to take children along to the demonstrations in order to avoid police intervention and to avoid contact with the press (di Miceli 2021). The protests were mainly organized on social media, and the promoters refused to inform the police authorities of the planned events, as is required by Italian law (ibid.). On 1 September 2021, the day the Green Pass became compulsory in order to use public transport as well as for entering schools and universities, the group (which claimed to have 40,000 online members) called for railway stations to be blocked in fifty-four cities, without, however, succeeding in blocking any of them. According to a police report on the group, 'The content and tone were exasperated, with explicit references to "hangings", "shootings", "kneecapping", as well as direct allusions to "new marches on Rome" and terrorism; among those identified there are also individuals who had promoted motorway and railway blockades as well as activists who have been involved in street attacks on the police engaged in ensuring Public Order' (Polizia di Stato 2021).

---

[1] A similar purpose was expressed by local groups such as *No Paura Day* ('No Fear Day'), active in Cesena, with a Facebook account that posted calls to take part in protests and pictures of their events (characterized by small groups of relatively older protestors).

Many of investigated activists were already known to the police forces, both for having adhered to extremist positions and for previous crimes such as resisting public officials, theft, robbery, extortion, and drug dealing (ibid.).

Another, competing, umbrella organization, the *Fronte del Dissenso* ('Dissent Front') aimed at creating a convergence of various groups under slogans such as ending the dictatorship and re-establishing constitutional freedom. Founded in Rome in April 2021, the organization saw the participation of various anti-EU groups (including splinter groupings from the Lega and the Five Star Movement) calling for 'national sovereignty' and the 'defence of the fatherland'. With a centralized structure, the *Fronte del Dissenso* presents itself as a unitary confederative movement which, in order to contribute to overcoming the fragmentation of anti-system forces, unites citizens, movements, associations, purpose committees, trade unions, and parties that agree on the claim that the Constitution of 1948 must be properly implemented, re-evaluating its principles of social justice, freedom, emancipation, democracy, and popular, national, and monetary sovereignty (Fronte del Dissenso 2021). As one of the speakers stressed during the founding event in April 2021, 'we need to go beyond fragmentation, the moment of spontaneity is behind us. From this assembly we hope to build a national coordination, from which we can develop a platform.' The Front claimed to stimulate, organize, and coordinate the various struggles of popular resistance opposing the attempt by globalist elites to build a new technocratic and neoliberal tyranny that implies the elimination of individual identity and of nations, as well as the dismantling of social rights and personal freedoms (ibid.). As it states in its manifesto:

> The Dissent Front declares its loyalty to the Fatherland and sets out to change the status quo, and to this end includes anyone who shares these premises, whatever their political and/or religious faith; it rejects the right-center-left classification, which has long become a weapon of the elite to keep the popular classes divided and subjugated, pushing them more and more towards alienating homologation and social subordination. (ibid.)

A further group that aimed to coordinate protests is the *Coordinamento 15 Ottobre* (AttoPrimo ODV 2021) which was created in the autumn of 2021 to promote a national mobilization. In its founding manifesto, the group claims to be opposed to repression, addressing the *Popolo d'Italia* ('the People of Italy') as well as unspecified *'portatori di interessi'* ('stakeholders').

As these attempts at action coordination failed, many protest mobilizations, especially in late 2021 and early 2022, followed a crowdsourced organizational model (see Chapter 3), involving local groups of anti-vax activists in particular, some of whom were directly affected by the policies of compulsory vaccination. Anti-vaxxers were invited to mobilize, mainly through online channels, with highly emotional appeals concerning the unjust persecution of those who were attempting to resist powerful plots. Thus, in a press release reporting on a flash mob carried out by suspended unvaccinated teachers in Florence, the CIL—*Coordinamento Istruzione per la Libertà*, INScdNO—*Insegnanti che dicono «NO»* (La Nazione 2021) stated: 'We are waiting outside … for the return of democracy':

> Left out like dogs from the places of honourable and fruitful work, even removed from social spaces, they distributed the leaflets attached here, addressed to the educational community in schools and to the entire citizenry, underlining:—the founding values of the Constitutional Charter (Art. 1, Art. 3, and Art. 32),—the objective data of the scientific literature (the vaccine does not protect against contagion),—the serious shortcomings of the public health system (the number of beds was not extended and the non-covid patients were neglected),—the criticalities of the therapeutic approach adopted by the Regions and the Government (the covid patients hospitalized in nursing homes; the lack of approval of home care, and the dissuasion from autopsies …),—the unjustified distortion of relationships between people (fomented by the media),—the pedagogical disaster that occurs in schools and universities (chicken-coop classes, understaffed personnel, remote teaching),—the unacceptable risk of administering an experimental drug even for the youngest population
>
> **(flash mob, 22–3 December 2021, firenze locandina scuola).**

During the second wave, most notably from the commencement of the vaccination campaign in December 2020 and the introduction of the vaccination certificate in July 2021, people identifying and identified initially as anti-vax, and subsequently mainly as anti–Green Pass, formed the core of participants in the protests (Figure 2.3).

The presence of actors from the far right, visible since the very beginning, remained quite consistent throughout the period in question, albeit with a gradual decrease over time. As early as April 2020, the neofascist group *Forza Nuova* (FN, 'New Strength') called on its followers to protest against the 'mass arrests of 60 million Italians' by a 'police state' which was taking the Chinese dictatorship as a model, and against 'Brussels and Beijing'. While some protests were directly organized by far-right actors, most notably FN and its Roman leader Giuliano Castellino, others were infiltrated by the same actors, at times creating tension with other protest organizers. Promoting an anti-gender discourse in alliance with ultraconservative Catholic groups such as Militia Christi or Pro-Vita onlus (Frazzetta 2022: 240), the group, which had already organized protest action during the first lockdown, against what it claimed was a 'sanitary dictatorship' that was exploiting a rather innocent virus in order to increase control over the population, was present in the main moments of escalation, from the fights with the police in Naples on 23 October 2020 to the assault on the headquarters of the Confederazione Generale Italiana del Lavoro, Italian general configuration on labour (CGIL) in Rome on 9 October 2021. Throughout this whole period the group promoted perturbative actions in defiance of the anti-contagion rules, in the name of the defence of personal freedoms and in resistance to the 'Great Reset'. In its call for a 'procession' to Saint Peter's in Rome to mark Easter 2020, in violation of the lockdown measures, *Forza Nuova* stated that 'Easter will be Christian', 'a day of struggle and prayers' (ibid.: 209). Isolated from the other far-right groupings and the far-right parties in Parliament, *Forza Nuova* subsequently looked for support by participating in protests organized by anti-vax groupings. Although the other, larger far-right group, *Casa Pound*, did not deny the danger posed by the virus and generally complied with the anti-contagion rules, alongside its programme of food distribution from 'Italians to Italians', it also organized weekly sit-ins (with social distancing and masks in the colours of the Italian flag) to protest against the limited government support to Italians in need. The solutions it proposed included nationalization and economic supports for both firms and citizens, while it accused the government of instead providing support for migration.

Both groups participated in protests organized by entrepreneurs, especially in the tourist sector, mobilizing with the network of restaurant owners *Io Apro* ('I open'), who challenged the lockdown and the curfew by keeping their shops open (ibid.). In doing this, they both built upon their previous alliances with the so-called *movimento dei forconi*, or 'orange vests', which had promoted road blocks and other disruptive forms of action during the financial crisis (to little success). These alliances had allowed them to address social categories within the autonomous, small bourgeoisie, which were particularly badly hit by the economic crisis and supposedly abandoned by the left. During this second wave in particular, tiny anti-EU parties such as *Italexit*, *Alternativa*, and *Ancora Italia* took the lead in many mobilizations, as is also shown by the video analysis.

While the first attempt to follow the call launched in Germany for a World Wide Demonstration (WWD) on 20 March 2021 in Turin failed, another call to transnationally coordinate protests was issued by *Basta Dittatura* on 24 July 2021, this time achieving limited success. Transnational protests remained very rare events, even though there was cross-national diffusion of slogans and symbols. For instance, the slogan 'We are the people' had been imported from the German anti-vax protests as early as September 2020, during the anti-mask protests in Rome, and references to events in Germany in 1989 were made in placards and photos. It is particularly noticeable that symbols related to the QAnon conspiracy theory were shared at many events, alongside calls for President Trump to save the world.

The forms of action

Given the heterogeneity of the actors involved, the *repertoires of action also tended to be plural*, including conventional and unconventional, peaceful and violent, online and offline forms. Anti-vax protests initially spread in the traditional form of a vigil or flash mobs, as static small gatherings that were the only permitted means of protest during high peaks of contagion. However, over time they developed into marches of varying size (Figure 2.4). As the two protest waves experienced their peaks and troughs, following the rhythms of the spread of the virus and the institutional policies aimed at controlling it, escalations took place in the face of police attempts at enforcing prohibitions on demonstrations and the violation of anti-contagion rules, which impacted on the number of participants. While there was a massive number of court cases brought by activists against the anti-contagion regulations, these tended to fail, as the courts confirmed the legitimacy of measures that had been introduced. During the second wave of contention, at a time in which the vaccination campaign was underway, there was a considerable increase in radicalization, which included hate campaigns on social media, calls for walk-ins at the homes of politicians and medical experts (or threats thereof), as well as the damaging of vaccination centres.

Protests sometimes emerged as *violent*, with an increase in more radical repertoires over time. *Radicalization* was present from the beginning of the pandemic in various forms of defiance of orders related to the protective policies aimed at stopping the spread of infection. The refusal to wear masks was viewed as an act of resistance, and conspiracy theories spread alongside anti-Semitism and a downplaying of the Shoah.

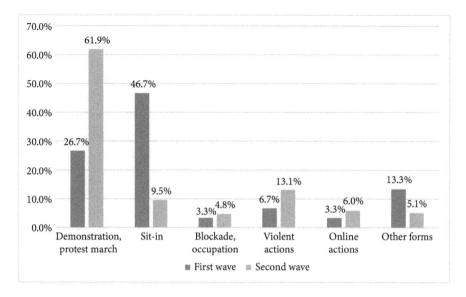

Figure 2.4 Forms of action by wave

Violent escalation had already developed as early as October 2020, during the protests against a new lockdown, which saw a particularly high level of participation by owners and workers in the tourism sector. In Naples, for example, protests started at 11 p.m. on 23 October against the establishment of a new night-time curfew. Fights with the police escalated in front of the headquarters of the regional government of Campania—as protestors built barricades, set fire to garbage and attacked police vans, while the police responded with tear gas and water cannons (Sky TG24 24/10/2020). As mentioned, in the same period, on 30 October, skirmishes between police and protestors took place in Florence at an unauthorized protest involving a few hundred protestors, who allegedly threw stones and bottles at police in riot gear (Sky TG24 31/10/2020).

One of the most violent developments to occur during the second wave took place at the national march held in Piazza del Popolo in Rome on 9 October 2021, at which organizers claim ten thousand participants were present. Roman salutes were observed being made alongside an abundant use of Italian flags, with activists damaging police vans and throwing chairs while the police reacted with baton charges. According to judicial investigation, these violent actions were led by leaders of the far-right party *Forza Nuova*, Roberto Fiore and Giuliano Castellino, who mobilized a section of the protestors to take part in an assault on the headquarters of Italy's main trade union, the

CGIL, calling trade unionists 'traitors', breaking into the building and damaging furniture and equipment, before trying to reach the seat of the Prime Minister (Il Fatto Quotidiano 2021).[2]

Further escalations occurred a few days later as a committee of dock workers in Trieste called a strike and blocked some of the entry points to the docks in protest against the introduction of the Green Pass to access the workplace. On 18 October 2021, the police used water cannons and tear gas to open access to the docks, with violent clashes ensuing between police and protestors, who subsequently occupied the central *Piazza dell'Unità d'Italia* and carried out protests in the following days, which often turned violent. Indeed, the protests against the Green Pass in Trieste received national attention, with 15,000 activists from all over Italy in attendance. One of the local union leaders, Stefano Puzzer, who had called for the re-establishment of privileges that the peace treaty signed following the Second World War had awarded to the harbour, became a national icon for the anti-vax protesters (ANSA 2021). In response to these events, protests were banned in city centres until the end of the health emergency.

However, most of the events did not involve violence, even if symbolic provocation through the refusal to wear face masks and aggressive behaviour towards journalists and passers-by were frequently reported. During the first wave of contestation, forms of action such as civil disobedience were also practised by some owners of restaurants that operated under the slogan '*Io apro*' ('I open'), challenging lockdown measures. In other cases, protests developed in more articulated forms, calling for the reopening of cultural and educational activities. Mobilizations against the closure of cultural activities and schools mainly took non-violent forms, including for instance the holding of lessons in the open air or students connecting to online classes from outside their schools.

During the second wave of contention, and especially in the autumn of 2021, protests were called every Saturday against the introduction of the Green Pass to access several types of buildings and businesses. Often, having only received authorization for static protests, such as *presidi* (sit-ins), the activists attempted nevertheless to form marches and to defy anti-contagion measures (i.e., wearing face masks and maintaining social distance). In order to reduce disruption to shopping areas (something that was often stigmatized by shop owners), from late November onwards protests began to be prohibited in city centres and the police launched investigations into episodes

[2] Four people were arrested during the protest; later on, a further five people would receive precautionary measures (among which, arrests and home detention), including three football hooligans and another leader of *Forza Nuova* charged with destruction and aggravated looting, violence, and resisting public officials (Il Fatto Quotidiano 2021).

of violence, in particular those against journalists.[3] The number of protestors, which had increased in October, tended to decline as time went on, while the police started to systematically identify participants at non-authorized protests, fine those not wearing face masks, file charges against those accused of resisting police intervention, and issue so-called '*DASPO urbani*', which banned certain people from accessing specific areas.

While a new directive from the Ministry of the Interior prohibited marches, on 14 November 2021, sit-ins were carried out in Rome, Turin, and Milan (the latter of which included a protest event organized by Robert Kennedy Jr.) but also in Gorizia, Naples, Florence, Padua, and Novara, among other cities. Participants attempted to reach symbolic sites—often under the slogan, widespread in the anti-gender movement, of '*giù le mani dai bambini*' ('hands off the children'), in response to ongoing discussions on the possibility of vaccinating children over the age of five. In Rome, a child was presented before a few hundred protestors as a symbol of children under threat, while activists from Forza Nuova called for freedom for their comrades in prison.

A further element that was imported from the anti-gender protests (Prearo 2020) was the narrative of victimization in the face of a supposed dictatorship that became prominent during this second wave of protest. As shown by the video analysis, from at least the summer of 2021, signs and symbols displayed at protests included swastikas, Stars of David, and striped overalls evoking those worn in concentration camps, all of which intended to imply a parallel between the persecuted Jews and the non-vaccinated. From as early as 24 July 2021, the words 'Vaccines set you free' written over a picture of the gates to Auschwitz appeared on posters in Rome, while in Genova protestors wore yellow Star of David badges to allude to their own 'persecution' due to their unvaccinated status. There were calls for a 'Nurnberg trial' to deal with the sanitary dictatorship, while the use of the Green Pass to access various spaces was compared to the Fascist era racial laws (HuffPost Italia 2021). On the day devoted to the memory of the Shoah, Israeli flags were displayed, marked with 1938 (the year in which the racial laws were introduced by the Fascist Regime) and 2022, or 1945 (the year of the Liberation from Fascism) and 2022. Extracts from *The Diary of Anne Frank* were read aloud to stress the similarities between the discrimination against the Jews and that experienced by anti-vaxxers (Giannoli 2022).

Given the declining number of protestors, in the last part of the second wave, more symbolic forms of action were employed. Towards the end of 2021 and the beginning of 2022 in particular, there was a rise in the use of

---

[3] In Milan, between 25 November 2021 and 9 January 2022, only religious, commercial, and cultural demonstrations were permitted to take place in the city centre.

hunger strikes on an individual level by schoolteachers who were personally at risk of suspension or were suspended as they either refused to show a Green Pass or (when vaccination became compulsory) had not been vaccinated.[4] In some cases, hunger strikes were also planned collectively. In particular, various anti-vax teachers organized a '*sciopero della fame a staffetta*' (rotating hunger strike) (Timpano 2022). In their statement, a group of twelve people undertaking a hunger strike claimed they represented the millions of people who were denied fundamental rights because they refused to obey state orders:

> We are a group of twelve people living in the Monza and Brianza area. Each of us will observe a fast lasting 24 hours in a sort of relay hunger strike that will begin on Thursday 3 March 2022 and end on Monday 14 for a total duration of 12 days. With this gesture we want to follow on the hunger strikes that began on 31 December with Professor Davide Tutino and was followed by Saverio Mauro Tassi, Diego Zannoli, Luigi Magli. ... The hunger strike is a definitive 'No' to an authoritarian system that has exploited and distorted the pandemic without addressing the problem of the lacerations inflicted on the social fabric. It is necessary to completely and definitively remove the segregation regime to which a part of the population is forced. ... We participate in the deprivations imposed on millions of people of all ages who, by government decree, have found themselves excluded from work, from social life, from free movement.
>
> **(Prima Monza 2022)**

Organizations were at times involved in the calling of hunger strikes. For instance, the lawyer Fabio Massimo Nicosia, president of the newly founded *Partito Libertario*, which emerged in the area of the Radical Party, announced a hunger strike to be started on 24 January 2022. On the organization's website, the hunger strike is presented as part of the non-violent tradition:

> This non-violent initiative intends to represent an antidote to the temptation to resort to violence, as this would in any case be legitimized by the principles in force on the right of resistance, Christian and liberal law, in the face of such disproportionate violence by the abusive power that is in place. The fasting initiative is also aimed at denouncing the one-way and discriminatory character of the major mass

---

[4] Individual cases are reported in the media, including a philosophy teacher in Treviso (Il Gazzettino 2022) or a music teacher (violin) in Milan who staged a solitary sit-in in front of his school (Fagnani 2022). In Rome, a philosophy professor was actually declared unfit for vaccination by a medical doctor, given his deteriorating health conditions following almost two weeks of hunger strike carried out in front of the government headquarters at Palazzo Chigi (Il Tempo 2022). Another philosophy teacher in Milan symbolically occupied his school against the government decision that required unvaccinated children to attend lessons online if an infection had taken place in their class (Bianchetti 2022)

media, as well as the censorship undertaken by social networks (Partito Libertario 2022).

In Verona, a hunger strike was promoted by a small firefighter's union (il Dolomiti 2021).

Between the end of 2021 and the beginning of the new year, there was also a wave of copycat collective actions involving the submission of formal complaints, filed at police stations and tribunals, against Prime Minister Mario Draghi, Health Minister Roberto Speranza, and other ministers (in some cases also the President of the Republic, Sergio Mattarella) for the crime of *violenza privata* ('private violence', art. 610 of the penal code) in relation to the requirement to display a valid Green Pass to access specific locations, including workplaces. These self-proclaimed 'mass denunciations' were registered in several Italian cities, where groups of a few dozen activists queued up in front of the police stations and tribunals to make their individual complaints.[5] During one of these 'Denunciation Days', activists were asked to use the texts prepared and circulated by a lawyer's office in Genoa that stated as follows:

> The vaccine blackmail imposed by the Government is not only illegitimate but in our opinion, it is indisputable that it constitutes a crime. The prohibition to work against those who do not wish to get vaccinated is equivalent to preventing people from being able to support themselves, their survival is threatened. It is a penalty that is totally contrary to the respect of the individual and human dignity, something that has never been seen in a state of law.

Denouncing what it claimed was 'blackmail' and calling for the judges to intervene in order to 'stop the authoritarian turn', the document asked that 'those responsible for the facts in the narrative, therefore the President Mario Draghi and the other Ministers of his Government, are punished for the crime referred to in Article 610 of the Criminal Code, possibly even in an aggravated form, or for those better seen and deemed to be inferred from the present narrative' (News Prima 2022).

Along the same lines, the Libertarian Party also presented an 'urgent appeal' to the administrative court (TAR) of the Lazio region accusing Prime Minister Mario Draghi and the Minister of Health, Roberto Speranza, of crimes against humanity, given their alleged persecution of the social group of the non-vaccinated (Porro 2022). Moreover, Codacons, an association that

---

[5] For instance, in Treviso (Tribuna di Treviso 2022), Bari (HuffPost Italia 2022), Parma (ParmaToday 2022), and Napoli (Crimaldi 2022).

was originally established to protect consumers, also put forward formal complaints against Draghi and Speranza, as well as former Prime Minister Giuseppe Conte, accusing them of 'crimes of attack on the constitution, usurpation of political power, criminal association aimed at subverting the constitutional order, political conspiracy and extortion' (Il Reggino 2021). Another campaign of formal complaints was promoted by the so called *Avvocati liberi* ('Free Lawyers') against Mario Draghi and the army general responsible for the organization of the vaccination programme, Francesco Figliolo, for crimes against humanity, kidnapping, crimes against the person of the state, manslaughter, procured alarm, and fake news (Rec News 2022). The *Movimento Fortitudo* also attempted to file formal complaints against Draghi and his government in Cremona, where, however, access to the tribunal was denied to the activists as they refused to comply with anti-contagion measures (Morandi 2022). The anti-vax media claimed that this campaign was a 'huge success', although the various initiatives were presented as being in competition with each other:

> Aosta, Arezzo, Como, Modena, Massa, Naples, Padua, even Lipari and many others: the complaints against Mario Draghi and Francesco Paolo Figliuolo are now rampant, they began in Bologna four days ago, with long lines of citizens going to deposit their complaints at the police station. According to some the non-elected (and apparently unwanted by most Italians) officials will not even see these complaints, because most of the naive dissidents—not all, fortunately—have filed the extortion complaint drawn up by the lawyer Marco Mori, in which the crimes cited fall under parliamentary immunity, while others are filling for 'private violence' which instead would have greater effect. ... However, it was a great success (di Mauro 2022).

Protests at the end of 2021 (Bufale 2022) also included calls to set the courthouse of Turin on fire as 'it is the den of the dictatorship that persecutes all opponents' (Famà 2022). The group *Basta Dittatura* published information relating to the home address of the prime minister, calling for a picket to be established there ('every night at 9pm'), as well as that of a doctor, Matteo Bassetti—without, however, actually going through with their plans of harassment (Gentile 2022).

Calls for roadblocks or railways obstructions, as well as the boycotting of the San Remo music festival, all failed. A roadblock proclaimed by a group of anti-vax activists—who allegedly called on supporters to 'throw Molotov cocktails at the TV trucks'—did not materialize (Open 2021a). Another initiative that apparently backfired was the crowdsourced creation of a map of shops and restaurants that were not asking customers for a Green Pass. The map, which was published online, was used by the police to impose fines on businesses and even to threaten them with closure (nextQuotidiano 2022).

Actions of harassment aimed at doctors and politicians were promoted by the ViVi (or Guerrieri ViVi, 'Living Warriors'), active on Telegram and Facebook, some of whose militants have been prosecuted for crimes, including the vandalizing of vaccination centres. In particular:

Coinciding with a peak in Facebook activity, the movement launched a 'ViVi challenge' on Telegram on 1 April 2022. The challenge called on users to post banners or graffiti with slogans containing anti-vaccination messages on official buildings such as hospitals. A scoring system was established to identify the 'best' vandal, taking into account factors such as the location and visibility of the banner. The 'winner' of the challenge was promised a cash prize of €10000. In the wake of the challenge, the Italian media reported on vandalism cases involving ViVi movement graffiti (Reset n.d.).

In the spring of 2022, the graffiti calling on citizens to 'Save the Children' were combined with those that railed against the 'Frauds of the War-Covid-CO2 Climate', perpetrated by a 'new Nazi World Order' to implement a 'WEF-WHO-2030-50 EU-ONU' and a 'Nazi–Communist dictatorship' ('the worst ever') (ibid.). These types of actions continued even when the street protests had subsided.

Expanding the comparison: Protesting in Germany and Greece

Although the degrees of mobilization differ in each case, both Germany and Greece have seen some similar paths of contestation of the anti-contagion measures as well as vaccination campaigns during the years of the pandemic, with peaks in protest following the peaks in the spread of the virus and related state measures to contain it. In both countries there was the creation of groups that opposed vaccination and episodes of radicalization within the protests.

In Germany, the so-called *Querdenken* (lateral thinking) protests started at a very early stage of the pandemic with the '*Hygienedemos*', organized in the Rosa-Luxemburg-Platz in Berlin on 28 March 2020, which although dispersed by the police was followed by similar initiatives in many locations throughout the country. Protests had already taken place before this in the south of Germany. In particular, the *Querdenker 711* group launched protests (such as the first one at the Stuttgarter Schlossplatz) under the slo-gan '*Mahnwache für das Grundgesetz*' ('Vigil for the Constitution'), calling in particular for the defence of individual freedoms. The initial prohibition on demonstrating enforced by the police, given the anti-contagion measures in place, was often reversed by the courts.

Since the very beginning of the pandemic, the impression of a rather heterogeneous base at such protests was reflected in the incongruent mix of symbols displayed during these events. The simultaneous presence of (apparently) contrasting references was noted:

> During the demonstrations, protest symbols could be seen side by side that could not previously be found at an event at the same time—at most on different sides during protest and counter-protest. In Berlin, a well-known Holocaust denier car-ried the rainbow flag through the demonstration, the black-white-red flag of Ger-man chauvinism flew next to posters referring to the resistance against National Socialism. And in Munich, neo-Nazis distributed the Basic Law... Above all, the historical references in the invocation of a 'Corona dictatorship' create common ground.
>
> (Teune 2021)

Indeed, the anti-vax protests have been described as questioning ideas long held by social movement scholars due to the unusual characteristics that they present such as:

> (1) The heterogeneity of the groups involved in the protests, from bourgeois Green voters to cranky hippies to staunch neo-Nazis. (2) The mixing ratios of these groups, which vary greatly from place to place, which do not produce a clear overall picture, but rather resemble a view through a kaleidoscope. (3) The diverse and sometimes contradictory use of symbols, which questions the usual attributions of mean-ing. And (4) the sometimes difficult to understand patterns of interpretation that drive the protests and prompted many participants to radically reject political institutions in a short space of time.
>
> (Teune 2021)

The choreography of the protests often also hinted at other waves of protests. In Leipzig, in commemoration of the events that brought about the break-down of the authoritarian regime in the German Democratic Republic in 1989, the protest at the Augustusplatz was to be followed by a march along the Stadtring. In a reference to the Montagsdemos of autumn 1989, the organiz-ers asked participants to bring candles with them, while pictures from 1989 were repeatedly shown in the video that called for the protests. The lights from mobile phones were used to imitate the cigarette lighters used in the original protests, accompanied by slogans such as 'in 1989 the East stood up, in 2020 Europe stands up' or 'We have no other choice. Out on the road, but it's going to be harder than in 1989.' In fact, according to participant observation at the event,

> The desired emotional connection was more reliably achieved through the repeated appeals of the organizers for participation and nonviolence. 'We are get-ting more and more!' and 'We want to create the fullest square that has ever existed here!' resonated from the stage before the official start of the rally to strong applause. ... 'Like 89! Exactly the same!' ... Through the announcements of the events as well as the statements on site, the promise was made that a 'historic moment'—that is, what will be history in the future—could be experienced live here. The proud shouts of 'We are becoming more and more!' as well as the cover-age in the various live chats of the movement testify to how historical significance should be created here together.
>
> **(Stach and Hartmann 2020)**

Converging on the narrative of an emerging dictatorship, anti-vax protests used slogans that called for resistance in the defence of Constitutional val-ues. In the initial protests at the Rosa Luxemburg-Platz in Berlin in the Spring of 2020, several participants brought the cover of the constitution with them, and distributed the version of the document printed by the *Bundeszen-trale für politische Bildung* (Hanloser 2021). The journal of the campaign Coordination Office for Democratic Resistance, known as '*Demokratischer Wiederstand*' (DW, 'Democratic Resistance') presented itself as 'loyal to the constitution', and against the anti-constitutional, terrorist measures of the government ('Merkel has to go' was a slogan that resonated with the mobiliza-tions organized by movements for democracy in the MENA region in 2011). The group claimed 'We are liberals far away from parties and dependencies. We believe that too many people are kept at home in mortal fear by the gov-ernment. The government is projecting its own panic over the collapse of financial market capitalism onto us, the people who have never had a funda-mental choice in their system as to how to set it up' (ibid.: 181). Thus, 'the protesters saw themselves confirmed in their own victim role in the criticism from outside, such as the reference to neo-Nazis and conspiracy narratives' (Teune 2021).

In the narrative spread at and during the protests, appeals to freedom and resistance were made alongside denials of the existence of the pandemic and/or fake news relating to its origins. As one study concluded,

> the official information about the virus is doubted and thus the pandemic situation is denied. The established media are criticized for their 'one-sidedness', as they would distort scientific facts or let the wrong experts have their say. The political-administrative measures are described as 'fear-mongering' with manipulative intent. Finally, the systematic generation of fear and panic is interpreted as a precursor to total surveillance and a pre-existing or approaching dictatorial control regime is lamented.
>
> **(Frei and Nachtwey 2021: 19–20)**

Indeed, the 'liberalism' of groups such as the German 'Democratic Resistance' has been said to mix postmodern philosophy with tolerance towards right-wing radicals. Fascism, instead, is considered to be a term that best describes the government, as 'Under the heading of Corona, we are witnessing the attempt at a terrorist dictatorship of the most reactionary, chauvinist and imperialist elements of finance capital' (Hanloser 2021: 189).

In Germany, as in Italy and in Greece, the appeals to the defence of the liberal constitution are at odds with the (broadly accepted) participation at protests of the far right, which provided organizational resources as well as a narrative. The national demonstrations in Berlin in August 2020 were already characterized by a very visible presence of the far right, including the main right-wing party, *Alternative für Deutschland* (AfD, Alternative for Germany). Subsequently, 'Local AfD functionaries often sought to take charge of these protests, which especially in eastern Germany were characterised by the very visible presence and participation of known neo-Nazi actors and their alliance with supposedly mainstream "concerned citizens"' (FES Friedrich-Ebert-Stiftung 2021: 4). While there was a strong presence of the far right in the protests that took place in the eastern states, it was not exclusive to this region. In Düsseldorf, as in many other cities in the western states, far-right activists (including members of the *Bruderschaft Deutschland*) participated in the protests. In general, far-right activists were often present as organizers, as were sympathetic musicians (such as the rapper Master Spitter) who performed at the protest events (Virchow and Häusler 2020). From the end of May 2020, the individual who was most frequently involved in informing the local police of upcoming demonstrations in Dusseldorf was a former Green activist who had subsequently moved to the far-right DÜGIDA (*Düsseldorfer gegen die Islamisierung des Abendlandes*). The relevance of the far right increased over time, through the three waves of protest singled out between March 2020 and 2021. The Far Right was, moreover, accepted by the other groupings involved in the protests. In fact, following 29 August 2020, when many right-wing radicals appeared at the second central Corona demonstration in Berlin, there was no condemnation of the Far Right

One of the most explicit examples of far-right parties providing the anti-vax movement with organizational support and visibility can be found in the already mentioned AfD. Within the party, 'The enemy images of an allegedly state-controlled "unified press" or "lying media" as well as "left-fascist" Antifa (anti-fascist) groups were also cultivated in 2020 in order to legitimize conspiracy-ideological, anti-Semitic, racist, nationalist and anti-democratic statements as acts of "free expression" and to stage the party as the patron saint of the "people" against a supposedly encroaching and dictatorial authority' (Richter and Salheiser 2021: 79). More generally, protest was particularly widespread where the Far Right was (more) deeply rooted; 'the legacy of radical right mobilization serves as breeding ground for the anti-system protests that emerged during the Corona-pandemic, particularly in the old states of Germany and for individuals that consider themselves right-wing' (Hunger et al. 2021: 2–3).

As in the Italian case, violence in Germany also tended to be especially widespread when protests were led or infiltrated by the Far Right. Among participants in protest events there were often a large number of AfD members as well as some of the party's Bundestag deputies, but also supporters of other radical-right parties, neo-Nazi groups, football hooligans, and *Reichsbürger*. They were particularly visible in an incident that led to an outcry among the public and in media alike when a few hundred protesters—many with visible extreme-right symbols—attempted to fulfil the widespread calls on social media to 'storm' the Bundestag, before being prevented from entering the building. As part of the event, 'At the Bundestag right-wing extremist demonstrators stormed the barriers, occupied the entrance area and fought with the handful of police posted there. Images of right-wing extremists waving the black-white-red flag of the German Empire in front of the Bundestag triggered national dismay on account of the historical symbolism' (FES Friedrich-Ebert-Stiftung 2021: 4). The very choreography of events in the summer and then autumn 2020 would seem to have been imported from right-wing protests in the US. The action repertoire also subsequently became more confrontational and at times violent, with attacks on members of the police and journalists, especially through the involvement of radical actors, such as individuals from the so-called *Reichsbürger* movement as well as supporters of the QAnon movement (ibid.).

Often, protests started peacefully, only to subsequently become radicalized. A demonstration in Leipzig on 7 November 2020, was described as follows:

> At least 45,000 people meet on and around Leipzig's Augustusplatz. In addition to conspiracy ideologues with QAnon shirts, evangelicals and right-wing extremists, there are anti-vaccinationists, freelancers, families. The mood is exuberant. One marvels and photographs special banners and costumes, the divided displeasure about the alleged 'health dictatorship' brings unknown people into conversation with each other. What unites those gathered is their conviction that they must stand up against an unjustified restriction of their fundamental rights. The fact that hardly anyone here wears a mask—for those present the symbol of an 'oppression' enforced by the Corona Protection Ordinance—is not negligence, but program. Although the organizers call for keeping distances, there is a dense crowd. When the rally is officially cancelled in the afternoon due to violation of the conditions, the demonstrators go to the inner city ring. It is black-masked right-wing extremists who break through a police barrier near the main train station and thus clear the way for the crowd. On this evening, thousands of demonstrators will once again parade around the Leipziger Ring. The police do not intervene.
>
> **(Stach and Hartmann 2020)**

The protests became particularly radicalized as the prohibitions on demonstrations were broken, with the demonstration becoming an aim in itself in order to demonstrate the strength of the movement (Frei and Nachtwey 2021). Furthermore, the presence of soccer hooligans from the beginning of the protests increased the potential for violent confrontations with the police (as, e.g., on 9 May 2020 at Alexanderplatz). In stark contrast to the calls for love expressed by the organizers of the protests, they often escalated into more violent forms. At the demonstration in Leipzig in November 2020, the organizer declared: 'You are brave to be there. ... Show me your love, show me your freedom. ... Peace Hey, Peace Hey, Peace Hey. ... You see that we are not a few. We are the center of society. ... Neither right nor left, I see people', stressing that 'all the world is watching' what he presents as a 'historical movement'. However, the protest escalated as the police attempted to disperse the demonstration; a few thousand protesters refused to leave and a group of neo-Nazis attacked the police, while others descended on the Inner Ring with candles, dancing to the song 'We are the Champions'. The radicalization in conflicts with the police became all the more widespread in the autumn of 2020, returning again in 2021 as the police started to intervene in a more decisive way against non-authorized protests and aggressions on journalists and politicians. Large demonstrations were organized in 2021, on 20 March in Kassel, 3 April in Stuttgart, and on 1 August in Berlin (using the slogan 'Summer of Freedom'), with an increase in the instances of aggressive attacks on observers, especially journalists.

A dramatic sign of this radicalization occurred on 18 September 2021, with the murder of a supermarket cashier by a man who he had asked to put on a mask (Benz 2021a). Indeed, the self-definition of anti-vaxxers as victims of a 'Deep State' justified the use of violence. Violence grew over time as:

> Self-stylization as resistance fighters and at the same time victims of a perfidious system has not only strengthened the cohesion between very different groups in the lateral thinking protests, but has also made the use of violence plausible and conceivable for many. From the very beginning, fantasies of violence and punishment have been part of the exaggeration of infection protection measures as a 'corona dictatorship'. While the use of force was initially imagined in the sense of self-defense, aggressive behavior and attacks are now becoming known from a large part of the protests. The targets are always journalists who document the protests, counter-demonstrators and police officers who have to enforce conditions or bans on gatherings.
>
> (Teune 2021)

Although protests were extremely rare in Greece, those that took place also tended to display a number of similar characteristics, particularly in terms of their development over time, the groups involved in promoting them, and the forms of action employed. As with the cases examined above, the protests in Greece tended to grow in number following a rise in infection rates and related anti-contagion policies. Additionally, the protests were organized by various different groups, with a significant presence of right-wing groups. In a similar fashion to anti-gender groupings in Italy, religious fundamentalism also contributed to the mobilization of protest in Greece. In particular, a number of protests emerged within the religious institutions. In spring 2020, Orthodox priests and monks attended meetings contesting the measures to reduce contagion. In December, with the death toll in the thousands, the Metropolitan of Corfu declared the Church 'under persecution', announcing that, in light of churches being closed at Christmas, the 'flags would fly at half-mast at churches'. Moreover, the Church adopted another very conflictual line over the feast of the Epiphany and the blessing of the waters on 6 January 2021, as: 'While the government announced that there would be no public religious rituals—in other words, the sacrament of Communion would be performed without the faithful—the Holy Synod (the supreme body in the hierarchy, comprised of all Metropolitans) decided not to follow the rules' (FES Friedrich-Ebert-Stiftung 2021: 6).

As for the more libertarian component, some events with limited partic-ipation were also organized by groups on the fringes of the anarchist milieu. The 'Initiative against the health Apartheid' formed in the late months of 2021 with a call to a demonstration against certain measures for Covid-19. More specifically, the group opposed compulsory vaccination, which they claimed was an unprecedented violation of human rights. Vaccination certificates were framed as 'certificates of health convictions', a reference to the certificate of social convictions historically issued by the Greek state confirming that a citizen was not a communist. In another document calling for a second demonstration, which according to reports mobilized 1500 participants in Athens, the group claimed that 'The imprisonment (*egkleis-mos*), the restrictions in movement, the prohibition of political gatherings, the lay-offs, the compulsory vaccination and the unprecedented violation of rights, are not characterized by [concerns for] healthcare but disciplining for the needs of the new normality imposed by the restructuring of capital, the overcoming of the capitalist crisis and the violent change of paradigm' (cited in Christou 2022).

Some protests also involved anti-vax workers in the sectors in which vac-cination was made compulsory in the summer of 2021 (all workers in the healthcare and education sectors, the police and the army, as well as citi-zens over the age of 60). Radicalization occasionally took place as protestors refused to comply with police orders to disperse.

Conclusion

This chapter began by describing the protests that took place in Italy against anti-contagion policies, disentangling the different waves that form part of a broader protest cycle, with different characteristics in terms of intensity, the actors mobilized, and the forms of actions, based on protest event analysis.

The analysis of anti-vax protests in Italy has indicated a number of trends, which would also seem to be shared with other countries. In general, protests were rather localized and small scale, especially during the first wave, with a few exceptions, especially in the second wave and in some specific cities. The rhythm of the protests followed the rhythm of the spread of the virus and related anti-contagion measures, focusing on lockdowns, the wearing of face masks, the use of vaccination certificates (Green Pass), and vaccination. In the first wave, claims were more negotiable, mainly oriented towards calls for public investment in certain policy areas (from tourism to schools). In the second wave, on the other hand, protestors more frequently denied the severity of Covid-19 and contested the very effects of vaccination, attacking vaccines as dangerous and denouncing the supposed existence of plots and a dictatorship. From a geographical perspective, especially in the second wave, the most numerous protests tended to be concentrated in a few cities, mainly in Rome and Milan, with some visible events also in Turin, Genoa, and Trieste (the latter all in the north of the country).

In general, protests were called by local ad hoc committees, with little resilience in the first wave, and some more developed structures during the second wave. In the first wave, employers and employees of those sectors more heavily affected economically by the pandemic organized protests against the second lockdown and curfews measures, with some escalation in cities such as Naples and Florence. In the second wave, we saw the dominance of various components of the anti-vax movements—from the exoteric wing to anti-Europe parties, from religious fundamentalist groupings to followers of various conspiracy theories. Far-right activists were present from the beginning, providing organizational support and bridging positions against anti-contagion measures with exclusive nationalism and calls for individual freedoms. During the campaigns, some coordination committees were also formed at a national level (such as *Coordinamento 15 Ottobre*, *Basta Dittatura*, and *Fronte del Dissenso*), which engaged in increasing internal struggles.

While episodes of physical violence were rare, protesters generally tended to defy existing rules against contagion and also verbally attacked journalists and bystanders. Violence was more present when the far right led the marches, or part of them, as was the case with the assault on the headquarters of the main trade union, the CGIL, in Rome. Street battles also escalated in Trieste, as some non-vaccinated harbour workers occupied a number of docks and the police intervened to clear them away. This led to the ensuing unauthorized occupation of the main square in the city, which attracted anti-vaxxers from all over Italy. Towards the end of the cycle of protest, there was a particular rise in attempts to use forms of action such as hunger strikes and formal complaints, which had only limited success, while calls for roadblocks or sit-ins in front of the private houses of elected politicians, experts, and journalists had no response.

In summary, the protest event analysis has made it possible to single out two quite distinct waves, which differ in terms of the forms of action and actors involved. In the first one, claims for public investment were mainly negotiated by collective actors, including traditional interest organizations and ad hoc grassroots groups. Indeed, the selective effects of the pandemic seem to have triggered specific grievances, which resulted in (at least partial) institutional responses. During the second wave, by contrast, dynamics of (not solely) symbolic radicalization were observed, with the convergence of anti-vax groups and far-right activists.

When compared with the German and Greek cases, we noted that protests had very different levels of intensity, with the former representing a case of high mobilization and the latter illustrating a case of low mobilization. This important difference notwithstanding, there were also similarities in the intensification of the protests following the development of the spread of the virus and related anti-contagion policies, the involvement of different Far Right groups in the organization of the protests, and their radicalization.

3

Organizing the Anti-vax Protests

A Disembedded Crowdsourced Strategy

Organizing the anti-vax protests: An introduction

The Coordination Group was developed spontaneously by teachers
and staff from the world of education who found themselves dealing
with the aftermath of this summer's decrees. It was born out of a synergy of previously active groups. In some provinces, we created chat
rooms, while in others they already existed. The logo was designed
by a teacher and there is a group that studies graphics and communication. There is a group that has organized an event that can
be replicated in all the squares throughout the country. There is a
group that studies the rules and legal actions. There are few rules,
and they are simple. Each province can change them as they wish:
as a rule, each person shows up in the chat, you must not write at
night, if there are too many messages, the slow mode is activated
(up to 1 hour in some chats) to allow for the participation of those
who do not have a lot of time to dedicate to it. … As an initial communication tool, open chats are created on Telegram on a territorial
basis. The groups are open to anyone who works in schools or universities within the specific area. To be admitted to the group, you must
communicate your name and surname and the institution to which
you belong. To improve communication, each group can introduce
other rules (night mode, limitations on sharing links and messages,
etc.). For the creation of each group, it is enough to have one person
from the area who acts as a link with the other groups. For organizational requirements, the representatives of each group meet as part
of a coordination group, which does not have decision-making func-
tions, but is instead focused on facilitating links and sharing between
the various groups.[1]

[1] Chi siamo?—Coordinamento Istruzione per la Libertà (wordpress.com).

Regressive Movements in Times of Emergency. Donatella della Porta, Oxford University Press. © Donatella della Porta (2023).
DOI: 10.1093/oso/9780198884309.003.0003

This is how the *Coordinamento Istruzione per la Libertà* (CIL) ('Education for Freedom Coordination') presents itself, in the 'Who we are' section of its website, as 'an informal project aimed at coordinating all of those who consider freedom to be an essential value'. The document stresses spontaneity and decentralization as the bases for mobilization, for which the group essentially offers chat rooms and easy to replicate protest formats. The aim of building a territorial structure is steered through the calls to self-organize in chat rooms according to certain guidelines. In a similar manner, various other groups offered platforms for people who felt they had been negatively affected by the anti-contagion measures, providing online instructions for self-defence. In this chapter, I will argue that the anti-vax organizational model can be defined as *crowdsourced* in its calls for self-organization, as well as *disembedded*, given its weak capacity for coordination.

As we have seen in the previous chapters, the anti-vax protests were organized by different types of organizations, from the Far Right to the so called anti-Green Pass and anti-vax groupings. While not identifying with one single organization, social movements are typically made up of networks of various individuals and groups, which are often also active in arenas other than protest (such as political parties, trade unions, third sector associations, squatted centres, etc.). In social movement studies, organizational choices have generally been linked to both material resources and normative preferences (della Porta and Diani 2020). Since the 1970s, research and theorization have stressed the importance of available resources in the environment, considering the presence of social movement organizations as a precondition for action. Social movement organizations are guided by strategic considerations as well as by *normative* concerns. The selection of an organizational model does not only follow rational assessments relating to the allocation of tasks, but is also constrained by existing organizational repertoires and assessments of appropriateness (Clemens and Minkoff 2004).

As they predominantly emerge during waves of protests, social movement organizations adapt to the specific needs of mobilizations in particular contexts, choosing from among a finite selection of repertoires of organizational practices. Formal and informal networks from different movements reactivate themselves or become more visible with every new tide of contention. However, cycles of protests also produce new organizations as well as organizational innovation (Tarrow 1994; della Porta 2013). This is particularly true in the initial phase of the protest cycle: as collective action tends to focus on the local level, mobilizations build upon grassroots groups that, although at times short-lived, nonetheless form the basis of further organizational transformation. As mobilization intensifies, the need for coordination brings about a proliferation of new networks. In adapting to the necessities of the moment, while at the same time reflecting upon past successes and failures, old and new social movement organizations are also influenced by new generations of activists (della Porta 2009).

Social movement organizations operate in complex arenas (Jasper and Duyvendak 2015) and different organizational models persist within any social movement or contentious campaign. While this plurality often brings about tensions between the different conceptions and practices of democracy embedded within different organizational models, cooperation also triggers cross-fertilization within broad social movement families. Moreover, as they are heavily influenced by the fluctuation of protest waves, social movement organizations are often short-lived, although at times they evolve towards associational models. Organizers also learn from previous waves of protest, developing solutions for perceived problems, with mutation occurring within organizations as well as in their reciprocal relationships.

While these general observations apply to very different types of social movements, research has noted quite different organizational models for progressive and regressive movements. On the progressive side, researchers have singled out horizontal and participatory models, characterized by loosely coupled networks—or networks of networks—with highly decentralized structures, based on symbolic rather than material incentives and fluctuating levels of commitment. Due to the fact that they grow during waves of mobilization, progressive social movement organizations have been influenced by the specific organizational taste of new generations of activists, with a particular focus on the development of participatory and deliberative arenas (della Porta 2009, 2020). An aspiration to experiment with innovative democratic practices has been observed for progressive social movements, who often aim to prefigure in their organizational structure the type of relationships they would like to extend to the whole of society (della Porta 2015). While the implementation of these utopian visions unavoidably falls short of the activists' hopes, they represent important references for any experimentation with new organizational models.

Conversely, on the regressive side, the widespread organizational model has usually been described as hierarchical, with charismatic leaders in competitive relationships with each other. While they are at times endowed with economic resources and powerful supporters, these groups also have a tendency to fragment and, given their propensity to use violence, to adopt semiclandestine formats. Subcultural dynamics have also been observed, often built around soccer hooliganism. A general hostility towards democracy is reflected in the organizational choices, which are nevertheless also strongly impacted upon by state repression and civic resistance against a conservative backlash (Caiani, della Porta, and Wagemann 2012; della Porta 2019). Far-right social movement organizations and movement parties that promote populist visions that seek to contrast the needs of the people with those of cosmopolitan elites, often defined in ethno-nativist terms, tend to maintain quite vertical structures with closed membership, well-structured organization and broad levels of power afforded to the leadership (Castelli Gattinara and Pirro 2018). Given the abovementioned connections between the Far Right and anti-vax protests, we might expect to see, to varying degrees, organizational trends like those described above for right-wing groups.

On the other hand, however, research has indicated new organizing logics that respond, in particular, to an increase in individualization, which we found to be especially present in the New Age, exoteric milieu. Addressing the impact of new technologies on organizational models of collective action, Bennet and Segerberg (2013: 13) have distinguished between collective and connective models. Large-scale access to social media offers interactive affordances to an independent-minded public (ibid.: 59) allowing for a shift in commitment levels, with individuals opting in and out of organizationally brokered collective action, organizationally enabled connective action or crowd-enabled connective actions. *Collective* action is the traditional form enacted by various types of formal organizations that invoke shared frames and mainly use digital media for communication and coordination activities. In *connective* action, on the other hand, media platforms are the central organizational hubs that allow individuals to activate their personal relationships. In this model, the acknowledgement of general trends of individualization and fragmentation pushes participants towards personalized paths of commitment through self-expression, which can be quickly scaled up through the involvement of a large number of individuals around personal action frames. The logic of digital media does not require organizational centralization, instead enabling the expression of highly personalized motivations. Technological openness allows for individualized networks. Within connective action models there is a further distinction between *organizationally enabled connective action*, in which a loose network of organizations mobilizing on an issue use digital media to invite supporters to take part in personalized action, and *crowd-enabled connective action*, characterized by 'dense, fine-grained networks of individuals in which digital media platforms are the most visible and integrative organizational mechanisms' (ibid.). Given the above-mentioned trends towards individualization, we might expect to find at least some elements of crowdsourced connective action in the protests against the measures aimed at reducing infection from Covid-19.

As we shall see in what follows, anti-vax protests emerged in what seemed to be a quite spontaneous manner, particularly at the onset of the pandemic, through local initiatives that involved tiny numbers of individuals. New groups addressed the different claims of the anti-vax constituency, ranging from the legal defence of those who had violated anti-contagion rules to media outlets spreading fake news, and from union-like to party-like structures. At the same time, however, the organizational structures of the protests did involve existing organizations, which ranged from anti-vaccination groups to far-right organizations. In terms of the development of the protests, while the number of protestors increased at regional or even national events, the mobilizing structures continued to remain quite thin, with calls launched on the internet, in some cases by little-known groups.

Although the anti-vax protests included groups of varying size and territorial coverage, as well as differing organizational structures, one of the main characteristics of the organizational repertoire they employed is what I call a *disembedded crowdsourced* logic. Generally speaking, crowdsourcing is understood as 'a sourcing model in which individuals or organizations obtain goods or services—including ideas, voting, micro-tasks, and finances—from a large, relatively open, and often rapidly evolving group of participants' ('Crowdsourcing' 2022). In the anti-vax mobilization, several groups presented themselves as a kind of platform, offering toolkits for self-organization. In this sense, the organizations provide services—ranging from templates for legal action to kits for the mobilization of protests—to an online constituency that is invited to use them. However, in contrast to the progressive anti-austerity protests that bridged a logic of collective networking with an individual aggregative logic (Juris 2012), in the case of the anti-vax protests, attempts at coordination generally failed given the weakness of the social rootedness of the pre-existing organizations.

In the remainder of this chapter, I will first look at a number of the organizational characteristics of this disembedded crowdsourced organizational model as it emerged in the Italian case. I will show, in particular, how movement entrepreneurs distributed resources for mobilization, targeting specific constituencies that they encouraged to self-organize. Consequently, during the pandemic and following the development of the virus and the related anti-contagion policies, anti-vax organizations aimed at catering to the specific needs of those who refused to be vaccinated, offering legal and medical support, as well as protest toolkits. While actions tended to remain localized, unstable coordinator committees (at times even in the form of political parties) formed in order to launch local protests in various cities as well as a number of national events. Resources were especially invested in social media campaigns that spread fake news relating to the virus and vaccines, as well as conspiracy theories concerning plots designed to deprive citizens of their rights or even to kill them in order to solve the problem of overpopulation. Over time, some of these fake news stories and conspiracy theories were reproduced across a loose virtual net, as they were propagated by the activists on various social channels. While attempts to build parties proliferated, these (mainly online) initiatives seemed unable to mobilize activists who, in spite of their regular calls for strong leadership, found none. The comparison with the German and Greek cases will show similarities in the crowdsourced organizational model, but also diversity in terms of the capacity of anti-vax groups to embed themselves in a broader environment.

A crowdsourced organizational model

In Italy, as in other countries, the protests against anti-contagion policy measures have seen the emergence of a large number of small organizations, which were often only active at a local level. Small nuclei of activists provided 'mobilization toolkits' to a constituency that they engaged with primarily on the internet.

Indeed, during the years of the pandemic, many groups emerged that followed a crowdsourced model to offer toolkits for mobilization online. In the document 'Obbligo vaccinale: Come resistere', the Movimento 3V (3V 2022)—a tiny party that adapted some of the ideas for decentralized organizing from the Five Star Movement—typifies this sort of personalized appeal to mobilization: 'We will not bend! Contrary to the plans of the ruling elites, you too can dedicate yourself to creating a different, cheerful, solid and supportive society, according to a human vision founded on the respect for life and the affirmation of the best in us: a society in which truth and freedom are the guiding principles in all fields of individual and social achievement' (Movimento 3V 2022). Thus, individuals are asked to self-organize and resist: 'The decisive tool for creating this society is a new political vision, in which you do not simply put your life into someone else's hands, but in which you know, understand, and actively participate in the decisions that build your society and our coexistence. ... With this awareness in our hearts, we respond to these new restrictions in one way: RESISTANCE!' Notwithstanding the conspiratorial vision of 'the plan to reformat society according to a transhumanist model', the group still defines its constituency as being made up of joyful and happy people. Thus, it instructs its readers to 'Network with all the free citizens you know, and look for others. Meet, identify each other, get organized. ... The real alternative to the brutality of this system can only come with a smile, with the desire to create and also to have fun ... and together this is far easier!' (ibid.).

The crowdsourced model is first and foremost used for the online provision of various kits for protest activities. Thus, organizations such as the *Coordinamento 15 Ottobre*—founded to coordinate one of the national protest events—calls for the self-organization of leafleting (Coordinamento 15 ottobre 2021.) in order to promote 'the big resolutive event'. Readers are, therefore, given detailed instructions:

> Print as many copies of the flyers as you think you will be able to distribute and donate them to those who cannot print them but are willing to help; If you feel confident enough and are tired of this situation, head to prime targets such as vaccination hubs, schools and day care centres; If you have a more reserved nature, you can instead go to parks or in front of supermarkets, swimming pools, gyms, bars and restaurants, public offices, public transport, post boxes as well as leaving leaflets on the windshields of parked cars.[2]

Formed around a splinter group from the Five Star Movement, the *Movimento R2020* also aimed at mobilizing on the basis of a crowdsourced model. Not by chance, R2020 presents itself as a 'container': 'a NETWORK of people united by the desire to reaffirm their rights of freedom, dignity and self-determination, rebuild communities of solidarity, protect the territory that hosts us, guarantee a happy present and future for all of us'. In this example the crowdsourcing model is connected with the self-organization of what the group calls '*fuochi*' ('fires'), which are defined as follows: 'A Fire is a local group made up of citizens, professionals and politicians who represent a territorial community: a town, a village, a municipality or the neighbourhood of a city'. However, coordination between these fires is very loose:

> The Fires communicate with each other to organize initiatives, campaigns and actions, thanks to the support of the professionals who have freely given their availability. There is no requirement to pay a membership fee: participation in R2020 is free. ... Since R2020 is a horizontal network and not a party, it is important to understand that there are no leaders, management groups or decisions taken from above. R2020 has no regional or national contacts, and is instead based on the coordinators of the individual Fires, who interact with each other.
>
> **(R2020 2021)**

---

[2] Coordinamento 15 Ottobre. https://fb.me/e/1Zr8nSQXb (accessed 30 October 2022).

Thus, the website promotes the self-organization of local chapters, for which the group offers certain tools—which essentially boils down to space on their website:

> Find a Fire in your area or start your own! ... Each local R2020 Fire meets periodically in a public meeting and decides which concrete initiatives to take forward on the basis of its priorities and strengths. Each Fire has its own autonomy and its own PROJECTS FOR THE COMMON GOOD. The national organizational network of R2020 will guarantee a space on the website www.r2020.it for each local Fire, where initiatives and projects can be uploaded, so that all of the R2020 Fires can share good practices.
>
> **(R2020 n.d.)**

The document then ends with the following invitation: 'Have you found a R2020 Fire already active in your area? Great! It's time to contact it! Click on the map and join your local group. You can also find an email address where you can contact the R2020 Fire representative closest to your home. Attend a group meeting and get to know other people' (ibid.).

Aside from the distribution of protest toolkits, during the mobilization against the lockdown and subsequently the anti-Green Pass and vaccination campaigns, several groups emerged that were characterized by specific entrepreneurial skills, especially those involving the legal and health sectors. In order to crowdsource the required expertise for their initiatives, people with specific skills were targeted on the website of the abovementioned *Movimento 3V*:

> We need you! If possible, we ask you to get involved in the project by first offering your contribution: Tell us about or put us in contact with anyone who has the skills to contribute. For the network to become widespread, we need you! With the same network spirit, we have started mapping every other profession. In the world of work that we are building, there is certainly place for you too! Doctors, lawyers, nurses, teachers, journalists, entrepreneurs, traders, professionals and workers with all kinds of skills can respond to our call.
>
> **(Movimento 3V 2022)**

As is also typical of other such groups, the toolkit provided by the *Movimento 3V* in order to promote mobilization includes platforms for the exchange of work and services ('If you need a service or manpower, on this platform you can find the contact details of people who will make themselves available to do what they are capable of doing'), mutual help ('The Ethical Professions portal brings together people motivated by ethical spirit, who are engaged in specific professions or who can make knowledge or products available'), production groups and purchasing groups ('Join or promote groups dedicated to local cultivation and purchase of food directly from producers who produce healthy food that you believe deserves to be supported. If you can, get to know mother nature by listening to her rhythms, or in any case by adapting your consumption choices'), babysitting and parental education ('Create parental and family schools or join the many existing initiatives. Team up with other families who are in the same situation as you. Exchange babysitting services with those in need'), as well as the exchange of books or car-sharing (Movimento 3V 2022).

With the passing of time, there was a particularly visible proliferation of websites and blogs in which legal skills were advertised, often by lawyers, aimed at opposing the various policy measures issued in order to contain infection from Covid-19. In some cases, the offer was targeted at specific constituencies (such as doctors and health sector personnel or teachers that had been suspended due to non-compliance with Green Pass and vaccination obligations) to whom individualized support was offered. Especially detailed suggestions were provided on practical issues relating to how to legally challenge state policies oriented towards controlling the pandemic. Thus, specific forms were distributed on the website of the *Movimento 3V* to be used to oppose employers or professional corporations who required their employees or members to be vaccinated ('If someone asks you to get vaccinated, in particular your employer or your professional body, we suggest you do as follows: download the following letter, edit the parts in red and send it by recommended post or certified e-mail to your general practitioner, forwarding it to your employer, or CCing them, for information'), to threaten doctors or public officials, to avoid paying fines related to lockdown violations, and to challenge the use of masks, quarantine, or the Green Pass. In relation to the vaccination campaign, the organization informs readers as follows:

What we suggest is an approach of active objection to impose compliance with informed consent, according to the principles enshrined in the Italian Constitution (in particular articles 13 and 32) and the precautionary principle. We have prepared three letters that can be customized and used in the manner most suited for individual cases. A letter of objection with questions (Letter 1)—A letter of request for examinations (Letter 2)—A letter to the general practitioner (Letter 3). We would encourage you to customize the letters as each situation represents a specific case and, above all, we do not want there to be any 'standard' answers. We believe that it is necessary for the objection letter (Letter 1) to be sent by those who have received written communication from their employer or from their professional body on the measures provided for by the Legislative Decree 44 (Movomento 3V 2022).

While most (indeed, almost all) of these legal complaints have thus far been unsuccessful, they enabled anti-vax groups to build ties with specific constituencies of non-vaccinated individuals and reinforce their choices. Especially, detailed information was provided to anti-vaxxers about how to interact with doctors. On vaccination, for instance, the *Movimento 3V* website suggests:

> All citizens, in particular those who are required to be vaccinated, must ask their GP for the prescription of the medicine (the Covid-19 vaccine); to all intents and purposes, the serums are, in fact, a medicine belonging to the National Health Service and a medical prescription is required for them to be administered. The general practitioner must perform a thorough medical history and prescribe any necessary clinical tests, the costs of which fall on the National Health Service (Legislative Decree 04/29/1998 no. 124), in order to assess the state of each individual's health.
>
> **(ibid.)**

Specific instructions (including a long list of medical examinations) are even given to those who eventually decide to attend a vaccination appointment with the doctor:

> If you decide to go to a doctor administering the vaccination: Ask questions about the safety of vaccines and the guarantee that there are no short, medium or long-term risks to your health. To ask your questions, you can refer to our *'I won't get vaccinated because'* campaign. Under no circumstances should you sign the free and informed consent form (without which you cannot be vaccinated) because, as you are subject to coercion, you are no longer free, and therefore responsibility cannot fall on you. Introduce yourself accompanied by a trusted person to act as a witness. Record the interview: You can record it without notifying anyone, but you must not disseminate the recording. You will only be able to use it for legal appeals or audio reminders. If you prefer, you can communicate the fact that you want to record the conversation. If the doctor refuses to continue the interview, ask them to write down their refusal and to sign it. If they refuse, interrupt the interview and document the incident by having the witness sign it. Use the document in any legal proceedings, lawsuit or appeal you decide to proceed with.
>
> **(ibid.)**

Another example of a crowdsourced model for the supply of legal services is given by the *Comitato Liberi Pensatori* which states that it is 'born out of the strength of free citizens, united by the desire to return to live in the most complete normality and truth, defended by International Human Rights and Natural Law' (Comitato Liberi Pensatori n.d.). On its webpage, the group offers links to specific templates that can be used for various types of legal action.[3] Similarly, a lawyer (president of the Libertarian Movement) and a trekking guide launched a website called '*Difendersi*', which provided templates to be used for formal complaints against the Green Pass and compulsory vaccination for health workers, teachers, police officers and other categories as well as an App to organize 'picnics to get to know each other' (Difendersi Ora n.d.).

Along with representatives of the legal profession, health workers were also involved in the crowdsourcing of expertise. Thus, the *Movimento 3V* promised to 'put at your disposal the network of doctors, operators and lawyers that, through collaboration and recommendations, it has created over time. If you need a doctor or a trusted lawyer, get in touch with your local contact person or write to the regional email account ... A group of activists dedicated to this project will help you find a solution' (Movimento 3V 2022). In the same direction, on the Ippocrate.org website, doctors and other health workers promoted alternative treatments for Covid-19 that lacked any scientific basis. Presenting itself as 'an association that mainly deals with research, prevention and personalized medicine, and which offered organizational support to a network of qualified doctors who provide free advice to people in need' (ibid.), the group states that,

> Covid-19 has highlighted and continues to highlight many contradictions in the modern world, not only in the medical and scientific fields, but also in the economic, social and financial fields... We have witnessed, to different extents in different geographical locations, the uncoordinated reactions of the so-called official scientific world: distinguished representatives of the medical sector, of the various branches of research, virologists, immunologists, epidemiologists and so on, often in contrast with each other, were however in agreement in opposing their other colleagues who, among many difficulties, in the field, sought a concrete solution in the face of the human drama and undertook certain therapies in order to save lives. The latter did not agree to leave the patient intubated, merely being administered oxygen only because there were no precise directives from above.[4]

---

[3] The readers are instructed to click on the chosen form and download it. They are also asked to sign and spread a petition against vaccination for children, which reads; 'Dear PARENTS, GRANDPARENTS, uncles, the siege continues in DEFENSE OF CHILDREN who, unfortunately, some parents are literally donating as GUINEA PIGS to pharmaceutical companies. This crime must absolutely be stopped!' (Comitato Liberi Pensatori 2022).

[4] Mauro Rango, 2020. '*Chi Siamo*'. Ippocrate.org, 14 July. https://ippocrateorg.org/chi-siamo/ (accessed 30 October 2022). Other groups operated in the same area, see e.g., Giulia Bertotto, 2021. '*Covid,*

Within the same logic of the provision of individualized services, trade union style groups were formed in order to cater for the constituency of non-vaccinated workers through the offer of online services. This is the case of the FISI, *Federazione Italiana Sindacati Intercategoriali*. In the 'Who we are' section of its website it reads: 'In a period of strong obscurantism, due to the virus that is gripping our nation, in which the freedom of choice and care and non-care provided for by the Italian Constitution is challenged by wicked political choices that impose obligations on non-contractual employees, only the "heretics" of the FISI have resisted the logic of the market and the powers of the pharmaceutical lobbies'.[5] Led by former members of the far-right groups *Casa Pound* and *Fiamma Tricolore*, the FISI has ties with the *Coordinamento lavoratori portuali Trieste*, several leaders of which have denied that the Covid-19 epidemic poses any danger and claimed that vaccines contain poison, while promoting national sovereignty as well as the claiming of extraterritoriality for the harbour of Trieste as provided for by the post–Second World War peace treaty (Luna Rossa 2021).

Another group which similarly bases its activities on a crowdsourced organizational model is the IDU—*Istanza Diritti Umani*: calling for 'natutal rights', it presents itself as

> a national association made up of doctors, health workers, socio-health workers and citizens, functioning throughout Italy with representation in every region of the country. The ever-increasing restrictions on natural and constitutional rights have forced us to unite to face up to the socio-political challenges and defend the fundamental values of humanity. Our main objectives are to re-establish impartial and complete information to the citizenship, protect the rights to work and freedom of care, speech and thought in the medical and civic sectors.

Promoting 'freedom of treatment' and denouncing vaccination as a 'mass experiment', the group calls for supporters to subscribe using a GoFundMe platform (through which it collected €390) (Istanza diritti umani IDU n.d.). In the same direction, Comilva (*Coordinamento del Movimento Italiano per la Libertà di Vaccinazione*) promotes 'active, conscientious objection' in order to obtain free medical treatment. On its website, services are offered (some of which are reserved for members), under the label 'Know your rights, assert your reasons', while outrage is expressed towards what they consider to be the

---

Grimaldi: *"Cittadini abbandonati mentre le cure domiciliari sono efficacy"*. RomaIT, 16 July. https://www.romait.it/covid-grimaldi-cittadini-abbandonati-mentre-le-cure-domiciliari-sono-efficaci.html (accessed 30 October 2022).
  [5] https://www.contiamoci.eu/wp-content/uploads/2021/09/STATUTO-9-settembre-2021-.pdf. ContiamoCi also operates in the same field (https://www.contiamoci.eu).

betrayal of the Five Star Movement and the Lega on the issue of compulsory vaccination for children (Comilva n.d.).

In summary, it can be seen that, in the Italian case, a crowdsourced model developed as groupings of different sizes used social media to encourage self-organization by distributing various tools for action online (from leaflets to templates for legal complaints). As we will see in the following section, this crowdsourced model remained disembedded, as a result of weak coordination within the anti-vax galaxy.

Disembedded crowdsourced organizational logics? The (failed) attempts at coordination

In progressive movements, as in the anti-austerity protests analysed by Bennet and Segerber (2013), the crowd-supported model of connective action is embedded in a fluid organizational network, which often proved resilient even after the decline of mobilization, as social movement organizations survived or developed into new ones (Flesher Fominaya 2021). However, the same is not true in the case of the anti-vax protests, in which attempts at constructing coordination would seem to have failed.

The coordination committees that emerged to organize protest events at a national level made use of social media as the main instrument for a crowdsourced model of collective action. This was the case of *Basta Dittatura* ('End the Dictatorship'), which was founded in the Summer of 2021 and organized a number of the protest marches that took place in the autumn of the same year, as well as very aggressive campaigns that targeted individual politicians and doctors, inciting anti-vaxxers to publish the private addresses of their chosen targets online (see Chapter 2). The group also advertised a number of roadblocks, most of which failed. *Basta Dittatura* was organized as a chat group on Telegram, where individual opponents of anti-contagion measures could converge and launch protest events, which often did not take place. The organization's Telegram account was closed on 28 September 2021, when the judiciary began to investigate a number of the members of the group for incitement to commit a crime, acts of persecution, aggravated threats, defamation, and harassment. In November 2021, following investigations in seventeen cities, the Italian police issued a report (Polizia di Stato 2021) that defined *Basta Dittatura* as 'one of the main web spaces within the world of Covid-19 denialists... the main centre of attraction for the organization of violent protests in the country... a principle node connecting the main web spaces for protests, characterized by a persistent incitement to hate and to the carrying out of serious crimes'. The accusations levelled against the group include having

> systematically called for the use of arms and for crimes to be committed against the main institutional leaders, including Prime Minister Mario Draghi. Moreover, some of their main targets have been the police, doctors, scientists and other public figures accused of being serfs and collaborators of the supposed dictatorship. Another group that is systematically insulted is the part of the population that has accepted to become slaves of the State by being vaccinated and respecting the rules.

Even after the original account was closed, similar groups re-emerged on Telegram (such as '*Basta Dittatura Ufficiale*') and continued to publish information on the private addresses and private lives of doctors and elected politicians (Open 2021a).

Another, similar but competing coordination body, albeit with a more political orientation and an offline presence, was the *Fronte del Dissenso* (Dissent Front), which aimed to create a convergence of various groups under slogans such as 'end the dictatorship' and 're-establish constitutional freedom'. Created in 2021 in order to call for a national protest on 31 July 2021 in Rome, the organization saw the convergence of various anti-EU groups (including splinter groups from the Lega and the Five Star Movement) that were advocating for 'national sovereignty' and the defence of the fatherland (see Chapter 2). The group largely complied with the rules governing the organization of demonstrations, such as informing the police as required by Italian law, while the symbols and flags of the participating organizations were allowed (di Miceli 2021). Participating in the *Fronte del Dissenso* are groups in the New Age milieu, such as *Alleanza Stop 5G* and a number of local sections of R2020, the party launched by the former Five Star Movement MP Sara Cunial as well as far-right groups such as *Ancora Italia* (a splinter party from *Vox Italia*), *Noi con Trump* ('We are with Trump'), restaurants owners organized in *Io Apro Milano* and *Io Apro Toscana*, as well as the World Wide Demonstration Italia. The *Fronte del Dissenso* has a more centralized structure than other groupings, which foresees meetings of the elected representatives of the organizations involved. It presents itself as:

> A confederative movement, which in order to contribute to overcoming the fragmentation of anti-system forces, aims at uniting citizens, movements, associations, ad-hoc committees, trade unions and parties that agree on the need to

implement the 1948 Constitution, re-evaluating its principles of social justice, freedom, emancipation, democracy and popular, national and monetary sovereignty. The Front stimulates, organizes and coordinates the various struggles of popular resistance, always in peaceful forms and under the banner of constitutional resistance, and opposes the attempts by the globalist elites to build a new technocratic and neoliberal tyranny that involves the elimination of the identities of individuals and of nations, as well as the dismantling of social rights and personal freedoms.

(Fronte del Dissenso 2021)

Another more short-lived grouping was the *Coordinamento 15 Ottobre* (n.d.), which was created in the autumn of 2021 to promote a national protest in Rome. Its main activity involved distributing leaflets, which in quite obscure language presented numbers from unknown sources stating that that vaccinated individuals pose a danger (they claimed, for example, that 14% of vaccinated individuals caused 64% of Covid-19 infections), that the virus is not dangerous 'for your children', and that Covid-19 test swabs result in very high costs for both individuals and society as a whole.

As the protests evolved, so too did plans to develop political organizations. The plan of creating a political alternative was initially addressed by individual activists. A shared element in these proposals is the idea of creating platform-based initiatives, which offer tools for self-organization and include explicit appeals to move beyond the Left–Right division. The (academic) activist Andrea Zhok, for instance, called for the formation of a political organization that would overcome the traditional distinction between Left and Right.[6] In a post called '*Cosa possiamo fare?*' ('What can we do?') (2022a), he promoted the idea of a front, cutting across ideological divides. As he stated in the post, 'there are not many glimmers of movement left', the only way to punish 'those complicit in this massacre' is 'to give shape to a political representation that is capable of competing for the electoral space with the current parties, therefore to a political formation capable of presenting candidates in the next elections and entering parliament' (ibid.). The lowest common denominator for this new political organization is singled out in the shared positions on the question of the pandemic. Therefore, while stating that the divergences in terms of traditional ideological backgrounds were overestimated ('I am quite sure that I would be able to find a great deal of common

---

[6] After the assault on the headquarters of the main trade union, the CGIL, on 9 October 2021, Andrea Zhok denied the influence of the Far Right in the demonstrations against the Green Pass in a post published on his blog entitled '*Alcune considerazioni sulla manifestazione No GP di Roma*', stating that all protests involve some level of violence and that the presence of neofascists had been used instrumentally to marginalize what he claims is in fact a massive movement (Zhok 2021d).

ground on positive political proposals with 80% of the individuals involved in this protest'), he suggested that:

> What is needed, first and foremost, is a united coordination of the multitude of groups, associations and individuals that have already mobilized against the government narrative and the subsequent regulations. This coordination must be established in an association of a primarily 'defensive' nature, which is not focused on the long-term aim of proposing structural policies, but rather on the short-term aim of restoring the conditions of democratic viability that have currently been suspended.
>
> **(ibid.)**

The plans for the establishment of a coordinated political organization relied upon the online mobilization of presumably self-organized cells. In the proposal put forward by Zhok, which is similar to those forwarded by several others, the main approach would once again be the provision of a platform:

> To give substance to this initiative, three initial operational steps would seem necessary to me: 1) it is necessary to have a proprietary virtual platform, an autonomous site, capable of performing some elementary functions; 2) it is necessary to collect, through this platform, the names of all those who in recent months have given signs of opposing the ongoing democratic degeneration (even through a symbolic payment, to be allocated to the maintenance and development costs of the platform); 3) it is necessary, working with the utmost transparency on the platform, to elect a certain number of representatives, who would thusly acquire the right to speak on behalf of the movement and therefore not simply as private individuals. This procedure can also be used at a later stage to define any applications. (Here we should discuss some technicalities to prevent possible 'sabotage' or 'hijacking' manoeuvres by organized groups, but more on this in due course.) In a subsequent phase, ahead of the upcoming elections, a phase of signature collection must take place to which everyone will be asked to make a material contribution (democracy cannot work only through remote clicks).
>
> **(ibid.)**

Similar plans for the creation of a crowdsourced political organization are shared by the leader of the Genova Libera Piazza group, which promoted the anti-vax protests in the city. Pointing to an urgent need for political engagement, he wrote: 'This should be condensed into a construction aimed at, nothing more nothing less, the formation of a new political entity that has the aim of representing dissent at the present and in future ... to try to get people into politics and into the institutions of the country.' Here, once again, the foundation of a party is planned based on a top-down framework that is expected to catalyse self-organization online. As he wrote elsewhere:

> I declare the need for the formation of an authoritative Promoting Committee, which is willing to publish an open manifesto-letter to a whole series of person-alities from the world of culture, work, business and civil society who are aware of and are active in opposing the regime that is being established, to stimulate them to take part in the open and transparent construction of the necessary political entity. … The people and associations that provide a positive response to this let-ter would form the founding and propulsive nucleus of the new Party—possibly not in a 'coalition', but as original constituents, thus avoiding 'reams' of differently ideologized acronyms with absolutely zero electoral appeal—, which would imme-diately set up its bodies, its procedures and its communication-reception lines for further support and content from civil society when deemed up to and consistent with the political-operational program.
>
> **(Franceschini 2021b)**

Another attempt at coordination based on a very decentralized structure, which emerged with the anti-lockdown mobilizations, *IoApro* ('Movimento IoApro' n.d.) was founded by the promoters of protests against the lock-down, lead especially by entrepreneurs in the tourism sector. Presenting itself (unsuccessfully) as a party list, the group aligned itself on the Right of the political spectrum, promoting neoliberal policies: 'Born in the middle of the first year of the pandemic, we were the first to make our voices heard, to defend our businesses and to be able to impose on the government the con-ditions and dates for the reopening of premises. Today the battle extends to all production activities and to those who find the adoption of outdated, absurd, inconsistent and discriminating measures to be beyond any reason-able interpretation.'[7] The core of the group's programme bridges the refusal of compulsory vaccination and the use of the vaccination certificate with demands for economic support for small businesses, as well as opposition to restrictions on the use of cash and against the '*reddito di cittadinanza*' (i.e. public subsidies for the unemployed) and the *ius soli* (an inclusive pol-icy towards migration) for fear that they might increase the rights of their employees, while at the same time calling for the introduction of a 20% flat tax. Also in this case, the organizational model is based on self-organization

---

[7] Indeed, a spokesperson of the group participated in the assault on the headquarters of the main Italian trade union, the CGIL, during an anti-vax protest in Rome in the autumn of 2021.

through meet-ups: 'Search for one of our meeting groups in your area. Take part in the demonstration, change the country' (Movimento IoApro 2021).

These attempts at promoting self-organization notwithstanding, there is a very pessimistic vision of their fellow citizens. This can be seen in the idea that participating in talk shows is considered to be useless as their 'audience is not ready to understand our reasoning, given that it is culturally and emotionally "loyal", if not to say "forced" by propaganda, to a whole series of issues and approaches that we have learned to call single dominant thinking' (Franceschini 2021).[8] Generally speaking, citizens are considered to be disinterested in politics as a result of a conspiracy developed by the elites to spread 'anti-politics', even within the movement itself. Thus, one activist stated,

> like the civil societies of the West, the alternative movement is pervaded by anti-politics, it no longer believes in its function … We must therefore understand that the demonization of politics was a political-media populist manoeuvre, favoured even within the intelligence spheres, in order to distance citizens from the institutions and from the political sovereignty of the country, which along with our monetary sovereignty was coincidently handed over to the Europe of the banks. This brilliant manoeuvre started in the period of *Mani Pulite* … and reached its 'splendid' conclusion with the Five Star disaster, which was in hindsight their greatest 'success'.
>
> **(ibid.)**

The commonly promoted idea of self-organization was also challenged by the very political bases that these tiny parties aimed to address, with activists taking to various blogs to complain about the lack of strong leadership. This desire to be guided is especially visible on the webpages of *Generazione Future*, in the comments under the documents published by the *Commissione Dubbio e Precauzione* (with the involvement of academics, led by the lawyer Ugo Mattei, who had previously been active in the campaign against the privatization of the water supply). While the published documents bridge a strong emphasis on the supposed democratic emergency with a denial of the efficacy of vaccination, several of those who engage in discussions on the blog promote more radical ideas relating to the danger of official science (as well as 'allopathic medicine' with some going so far as to deny the existence of the pandemic), and calls for instructions for action that they expect to be provided in a top-down fashion. Thus, in a comment under the

---

[8] Also published on Attivismo.info and Sfero.

'*Nota del 2 gennaio 2022. Sul dovere di difendere lo stato costituzionale*' by the *Commissione Dubbio e Precauzione*, a contributor stated:

> Like others, I too feel that I am in an ever-shrinking cage and I have the urge to do something, but what? We lack coordination, we must gather the support of magistrates, academics, suspended personnel: law enforcement agencies, doctors, teachers, the victims of vaccines who have been abandoned by the state … We must civilly disobey and boycott those who discriminate against us through the use of the Green Pass, as well as advocating this cause to awaken everyone's conscience. Lead us, we are here!
>
> **(Generazioni Future 2022c)**

Similarly, in the comments under the document '*Sulle misure "di contenimento dell'epidemia" adottate dal governo il 29/12/21*', one reader observes: 'Enough words … but someone must tell us how to act and give us a starting signal for disobedience … in this way we all end up becoming slaves forever …. A Revolution can be the only solution … but we need a guide … We citizens have been totally left to our own devices' (Dipartimento Giuridico Generazioni Future 2021).

In general, it can be seen that attempts at coordination had little resonance, with coalitions that formed for specific national mobilizations seemingly unable to survive in the long term. As has been seen to be the case in the anti-gender sphere, the proliferation of names for groupings often did not correspond to the presence of real organizational structures. The appeals to crowdsource did not resonate among followers, who instead called for strong leaders.

Remobilizing: From anti-vaccination to anti-EU and the Far Right

As is common in waves of protest, mobilization around anti-vax positions is also promoted by previously existing organizations. In particular, I have drawn attention to the convergence of the Far Right with a New Age milieu, which had already undergone transformations prior to the pandemic. Among the main sets of organizations that remobilized previously existing groups against compulsory vaccination for children and the related support for homeschooling are ultraconservative Catholics and the Far Right, which includes groups promoting national sovereignty against globalization. Some of these groups had already come together during previous anti-vax protests as well as in the so-called anti-gender protests, although the mobilized bases were relatively small and relations were quite loose. While in these cases the organizational structure tended to be more formalized, their coordination capacities remained weak as the crowdsourced connective model of collective action failed to embed itself in a dense organizational network.

A number of the groups that emerged from previous anti-vax protests had been involved in campaigns against the vaccination of children, in favour of homeschooling and free choice in relation to medical treatments. During the 1990s, associations for free vaccination emerged, especially in Veneto and South Tyrol. The claim about the recognition of vaccine damages was followed by the accusation of political-economic interests related to vaccination due to the Tangentopoli scandals, with a rehearsal in 2017, when a new law made ten pediatric vaccinations mandatory to qualify for access to elementary school. Groups such as Corvela and Comilva that originated in the earlier mobilization, during the Covid-19 pandemic immediately began spreading doubts on the effects of vaccines, which they accused of creating new variants (Morsello and Giardullo 2022). Vaccine sceptics expressed strong mistrust not only in Big Pharma but also in mainstream medicine as well as political institutions, promoting support instead for natural remedies, homoeopathic medicines and anthroposophical approaches (Lello, Bertuzzi, Pedroni, and Raffini 2022). Many in the *Movimento 3V* had experience in organizations that contested compulsory vaccinations.

Asking for freedom from vaccination, Comilva, which had organized a large demonstration in Pesaro on 8 July 2017 against the government decision to increase the number of compulsory vaccines for children aged from 4 to 10, presents its mission as oriented 'to support families who decide to practice conscientious objection, to provide medical and legal assistance to the victims of vaccines, to campaign for a change in the laws in force and to raise awareness of the issue' (Comilva n.d.). Calls against compulsory vaccination for children were also issued by the *Coordinamento Internazionale delle Associazioni a Tutela dei Diritti dei Minori*, founded in 1999, which presents itself as 'A body of non-profit voluntary associations, and of people and citizens who operate in the field of protection of the rights of minors, the family, and related issues' (Bocci 2019).[9] It had been especially involved in mobilizing against the compulsory vaccination of children, which it defined as

a provision against which, for two years, thousands of people have been demonstrating throughout Italy, which has closed the doors of kindergartens in the face

---

[9] In Commento all'articolo su Repubblica.it 01/04/2019 by Michele Bocci,

of very healthy children who have been separated from one day to the next from their classmates and teachers who, in some cases, even relegated them to sepa-rate rooms, where they had to eat in isolation because they were considered to be 'plagued' by certain zealous headmasters, and whose health data were even posted, in one case, on the door of the school. This is a measure that led to the closure of many schools due to a collapse in enrolment numbers.

(Comilva n.d.)

Organizations for freedom of medical treatment, which had been founded during previous anti-vax campaigns, also remobilized. Among these, the *Associazione studi e informazioni sulla salute* (AsSIS) presents itself as being made up of 'Doctors, health professionals, and lawyers who, in absolute respect of the principles on which their professional associations were founded, wish to work together with conscious citizens'. In a document entitled '*Green-pass e obblighi vaccinali per covid non hanno fondamento sci-entifico*' (AsSIS 2022), the AsSIS stated that 'The scientific reasons behind the obligation for vaccination and the restrictive measures of the Green Pass are based on the assumption that vaccination prevents transmission to oth-ers, causing a "pandemic of the unvaccinated". The scientific literature says differently.'

The attempt by the Far Right to use issues relating to vaccination in order to organize protests—including violent protests—was particularly noted by the COSPASIR Parliamentary Committee in its 2021 report (Cospasir 2021). This involvement can be located within the evolution of the Far Right in Italy. Prior to the pandemic, the Far Right had already been characterized by frag-mentation, with the two largest neofascist groupings, *Casa Pound* and *Forza Nuova*, developing along divergent lines. This can particularly be seen in the fact that while *Casa Pound* made a greater use of disruptive forms of action and built electoral alliances, *Forza Nuova* (FN) radicalized its repertoire of action and became increasingly isolated, also from the main right-wing par-ties, the League and Brothers of Italy. The pandemic prompted change, espe-cially in FN, which was already experiencing an organizational crisis. After the investigations carried out into a number of its leaders for violent crimes, including the formation of a terrorist organization, FN started a process of completely overhauling its symbols and communication outlets. During the pandemic the group promoted a new party, named *Italia Libera*, that claimed to be against the 'sanitary dictatorship'. In announcing its participation in the protests launched in the autumn of 2020 by emerging anti-vax groups, FN wrote of 'a broadening front, more and more plural, anti-ideological and popular, that sees the participation of men of culture and popular factions, freelancers and shopkeepers, football ultras and activists from different backgrounds, MPs and members of regional governments. All ready to overcome the old frameworks, the right and the left and build resistance' as 'in this dark time ... many are opening their eyes' (Frazzetta 2022: 212).

An alliance was built in particular with the *Popolo delle Mamme* ('People of the Mothers'), which bridged opposition to anti-contagion measures with anti-gender positions, as well as with other anti-vax groups such as R2020. These strands converged on 5 September 2020 during the national march in Rome and with the launch, a month later, of *Italia Libera*, as a party that aimed to unite Italians in the resistance against what they called the 'global Great Reset' and a 'Unified Covid Party'. *Italia Libera* was, therefore, presented as 'a union of dissident intellectuals, freelance professors and professionals, anti-mainstream scientists, citizens, antagonists, workers, autonomous workers, precarious individuals and students from all backgrounds converging today on a single and unique goal: a Free Italy' (ibid.: 214). *Forza Nuova* then announced its decision to enter into a single great team with the orange vests and the anti-mask universe: '*Forza Nuova* is the movement of the revolution. Today it opens up space to the larger and variegated *Italia Libera* because it understands that it cannot defeat the obstacle of the sanitary dictatorship alone .... Our program persists but pragmatic reasons push us to take the lead in a larger movement that is capable of achieving the chosen aims' (ibid.: 244). While stating that they did not want to dissolve their own party as part of this experience, in May 2021, *Forza Nuova* promoted *Area*, as a 'movement of movements' in which all fascist groups were called upon to converge.

Within this milieu, a section of anti-vaccination activists is rooted in the most conservative segments of the Catholic Church, in groups that had already mobilized against abortion and for a Christian Italy, denouncing Pope Francis as the anti-pope and proclaiming their loyalty to his predecessor, Benedict XVI. Thus, for instance, the website of the *Coordinamento Nuova Influenza* (@Coordinamento15ottobreripristinato) hosted comments from seemingly very religious supporters who state 'I pray to the Lord every day', 'May God enlighten your mind, guide your actions, make you strong, patient, persevering'. Elsewhere, on Visione TV, there were denunciations against the 'character assassination' of Benedict XVI (Sartori 2022).

Posters that were regularly displayed against face masks for children or the vaccination of minors read '*I bambini non si toccano*'[10] ('Hands off our children')—a slogan broadly used by the anti-gender movement. Indeed, groups active against gender rights that had split from the broader 'For the

[10] https://www.facebook.com/Coordinamento15ottobreripristinato/ (accessed 30 October 2022).

Family' campaign organized within the Catholic Church also remobilized from previous campaigns against the vaccination of children. Within the Italian context, the anti-gender network emerged in 2013, as the result of a split within the pro-life movement. The most conservative part of this milieu shifted their focus from family support to the opposition of 'gender', which they conceived to be a challenge to the traditional vision of sexually determined roles. While proclaiming a willingness to go beyond the Catholic reference base, the anti-gender groupings continued to meet in parishes and enjoyed a certain level of informal support from bishops. However, following the model of the French *Manifs pour tous*, the anti-gender movement developed as an attempt to gain autonomy from the Church (which they saw as overly oriented towards compromise) and to instead acquire the support of far-right parties and leaders for their ultra-conservative aims (Lavizzari 2021). The call to protect children (which not by chance is at the core of the QAnon conspiracy and was broadly used during anti-vax protests during the Covid-19 pandemic) was one of their central messages, reported in the very name of the national coordination body of the *Comitato difendiamo i nostril figli* ('Committee to defend our children') as well as in the names of groupings such as the *Comitato di mamme ce n'è una sola* (There is Only one Mom Committee). While the party that emerged from within the anti-gender milieu, the *Popolo della famiglia* (the People of the Family), repeatedly failed to garner electoral support, the anti-gender campaign was successful in building an alliance with far-right parties such as the Lega and Brothers of Italy. While the Far Right saw in the anti-gender movement the possibility to expand their electoral base, the anti-gender campaign provided their politicians with religious symbols of identification (such as crucifixes and rosaries). Although support for life (from conception to natural death) was still a central issue, the main targets became the rights of women and the LGBTQ community, with protest opposing not only assisted procreation or same-sex marriage, but also laws against homophobia and transphobia. Some of these grouping had already networked with the right-wing and anti-vax milieus on parental education, claiming full freedom for parents in the education of their children, thus bridging the protection of the 'natural family' with exclusionist concepts of national sovereignty. In this milieu, for instance, the *Popolo delle mamme*, which focuses on homeschooling, participated in anti-vax protests organized by the right-wing party *Ancora Italia*.

Within the anti-gender movement, another set of existing groups that mobilized in support of the anti-vax cause were those defending the proclaimed rights of fathers, which they consider to be under attack from feminism. Opposing the Green Pass, in its 'Manifesto' (La Fionda n.d.), the group *La Fionda* bridges appeals for freedom of expression with statements against 'gender theory', stating: 'There are only two genders, corresponding to the two sexes defined by genetic heritage: i.e. male, typical of men, and female, characteristic of women.' An extremely virulent anti-feminist discourse is thus connected with anti-vax positions:

> The denigration of the male gender and its arbitrary and unfounded description as violent, aggressive, inhuman and insensitive, as a subject not worthy of being understood in its needs and desires, in its right to happiness and in its humanity, nor worthy to be appreciated and valued for its merits and excellence, and therefore as fully expendable or secondary, is a mystification … imposed by a permeating ideological and destructive extremism, which draws benefits, privileges, power and resources from the indiscriminate blaming of the male gender, from the consequent conflict between men and women, and from the destruction of their common regulatory agencies, above all the family. Feminism, which falsely claims to fight for equality between men and women against an alleged 'patriarchal regime', actually wages a war of annihilation on the figures of man and the father, with the aim of acquiring privileges, primacy and advantages for an ideologized minority that defines itself as the representative of an entire community characterized by gender. In openly considering the male half of the world an enemy that must be fought, feminism is the greatest cause of imbalance and the greatest obstacle to achieving full and harmonious equality between men and women.
>
> (ibid.)

Several of the groupings supporting the anti-vax protests had also emerged during previous anti-EU campaigns, mainly conducted on the Far Right, within which they had not only collaborated but also competed. In this environment, anti-EU rhetoric was bridged with increasingly conspiratorial views on Covid-19 by *Liberiamo l'Italia*, an anti-EU group which has been a main promoter of one of the organizations that coordinated anti-vax protests, the abovementioned *Fronte del Dissenso* (their original Manifesto stated, 'Let's escape from the EU cage, take back sovereignty by regaining democracy'). Founded in 2019 with the proclaimed aim of defending the 1945 Italian Constitution against the EU, through the creation of *Comitati Popolari Territoriali* (Local People's Committees), the group subsequently presented itself as a central nucleus for an emerging anti-vax party (Liberiamo L'Italia 2022). Similar positions are promoted by the far-right party *Casa Pound*.

There are several examples of common initiatives among the groups mentioned here. For instance, the *Associazioni per la Tutela dei Diritti dei Minori*

(C.I.A.T.D.M), along with the with *Coordinamento 15 Ottobre, ContiamoCi!* and the *Associazione di Studi e Informazione sulla Salute* (AsSIS) signed a press release to promote legal complaints against institutional figures for crimes against humanity due to their support for the measures on vaccination (Coordinamento 15 Ottobre 2022). The anti-EU, far-right party *Ancora Italia* (whose leaders come from a split in Vox Italy, a far-right, anti-EU party) called for a protest in Milan: 'Together with the *Popolo delle mamme* (People of the Mothers), the LES union of the State Police and other groups, movements and associations similar to us in fighting this sanitary dictatorship. Only unity in the struggle can save us from this sanitary dictatorship' (Visione TV 2022).

However, previous ties notwithstanding, these attempts at building long-lasting coalitions failed. At the 2022 parliamentary elections, the presence of six electoral lists testifies to the intense internal competition that existed, which was also often fuelled by personal animosity. The failure of attempts at organizational structuration is also indicated by the fact that none of these party lists succeeded in electing any representative, while (confirming the regressive political alignment of the anti-vax protests) some anti-vax MPs were elected in the lists of the Brothers of Italy and of the League.

Communicating fear: The social media net

An important coordination function within the anti-vax net was played by the many social media outlets that were developed. They shared fake news relating to the virus and vaccination as well as attempting to constructing positive symbols (i.e. anti-vax celebrities and those who had died unvaccinated and were praised as heroes). Through the spreading of conspiracy content, various types of social media accounts aimed to create a virtual net, connecting various types of outlets. Both journalists and communication experts provided specific communication skills in this effort, which was also based upon a crowdsourced model, in terms of both its financing and its organization, oriented as it was to collect content from users as well as self-appointed experts. While the number of blogs, websites, Facebook accounts, Telegram channels, and YouTube Channels involved was very high, the connections between them remained weak.

An element that is common to all of these communication outlets is that they present themselves as defenders of a freedom of expression they consider to be under attack. Claims for freedom of information were issued by the main coordination channels of communication, TV Byoblu, which hosts speeches from representatives of the various anti-vax groups, functioning as a sort of hub (in Becchi 2021). Founded in 2008 as the blog of Claudio Messora, a journalist who later became a communications consultant for the Five Star Movement (which subsequently distanced itself from him), Byoblu is among the websites that were accused by Google of spreading fake news and banned from using AdSense, the platform for online advertising (Rovelli 2017). In attacking the decision, the journalist claimed that it was part of a conspiracy organized by Hillary Clinton, the European Parliament, and Angela Merkel, among others. Similarly, Visione TV declares itself to be devoted to 'defending freedom of thought and expression, which today more than ever are threatened by the single thought imposed on us by a prevalent media system that has lost any sense of limits and measures. Helping citizens to independently develop critical thinking on the things that happen in Italy and in the world is our mission' (Visione TV n.d.).

While the degree of denial of the existence of a pandemic and the support for a vision of global conspiracies vary along with the communication style, which has a wide range of sophistication and professionality and caters for different audiences, the content that was shared mainly refers to the assumed dangers of vaccination and the mildness of the Covid-19 virus as well as plots involving the elite relating to the pandemic. In general, these media outlets often posted and reposted fake news that increased fear in relation to vaccination as well claims of a supposed global plot aimed at literally killing a large part of the population (their estimates vary from 50% to as much as 90% of the world) as well as to subjecting them to total domination. In this fashion, specific fake news stories as well as texts illustrating various conspiracy theories were published online by various channels of communication.

The various media channels shared a narrative of victims and heroes, posting pictures of anti-vax protesters and supposed victims of vaccination. Moreover, several prominent anti-vax activists who died of Covid-19 (in some cases due to the fact that they refused to receive treatment) essentially assumed the mantle of martyrs, as was the case for a biologist who had founded the organization *Uniti per la Libera Scienza* and participated in various TV and radio programmes (Spica 2022). Some of the national and international icons most often mentioned those few scientists who adopted anti-vax positions. Thus, for instance, the online TV channel Telecolor Greenteam posted interviews with anti-vax icons as well as their biographies. In addition to this, the statements of self-proclaimed counter-experts were both cited and circulated. The website of the media outlet *Cataniattiva* placed great emphasis on its reporting of the statement by the Nobel Prize winner Michael Levitt, who was said to consider Covid-19 to be a normal virus (Catania Creattiva 2022). On another website, *Il Paragone*, the 'renowned and very respectable scientist', Professor Christian Perronne, is reported as giving a speech at the 'European Parliament in Luxemburg' (a point that confuses Strasbourg with Luxembourg and the European Parliament with the Parliament of Luxembourg), in which he stated that 'Officially we now know that this vaccine has already killed 36000 people in Europe, 25000 in the United States, including hundreds of athletes, as well as a large increase in cancer deaths after vaccination. The best example is that the countries that have not vaccinated their populations or have stopped vaccinating are those in which the epidemic has ended' (Giulia 2022).

In particular, QAnon narratives were bridged with vaccination refusal for instance on *Conoscenze al confine* (Knowledge at the Border), a website that publishes content on alternative medicine, yoga and esotericism, among other topics (https://www.conoscenzealconfine.it/). Fake news published on the website included the following:

> the Covid-19 test implant 'Darpa hydrogel' (an 'artificial substance acting as a converter between the electromagnetic signal and the living cell, tissue and organ'); the presence of graphene in Covid vaccines, which connects to 5G networks; the presence of self-replicating parasites in Covid vaccines, which are seen as the first step of the introduction of a new species of human android; deaths of airplane pilots hidden by official sources and mainstream media; side effects of vaccines in the circulatory system; magnetism in vaccines; the Marburg virus and next pandemic; cyber-pandemic and the so-called Big Reset.
>
> **(Murru 2022)**

As recently as January 2023, the website published a post stating that the WHO had launched a war against the non-vaccinated, who they considered to be 'murders'. Consolidating the narrative of a dictatorship, the activists denounces the corruption and the complicity of the public health system as a 'global Covid coup d'etat'.[11] In general, it has been noted that populist communicators often claim to develop 'counterknowledge', professing a belief in truth achievable by inquiry supported by alternative experts (Ylä-Anttila 2018). Indeed, on several anti-vax outlets the communication style tends to imitate a scientific tone. As has been noted for the *Conoscenze al confine* website,

> In each of the considered articles, there is a recursive scheme: a revelation of facts and numbers that are hidden by the entire establishment (including media, politicians and mainstream scientists) and that prove that all medical and restrictive

---

[11] https://www.conoscenzealconfine.it/oms-nel-2023-guerra-ai-non-vaccinati-definiti-assassini/

measures taken by the government to control the pandemic will be used to secretly destroy humankind or transform part of it into a mass of enslaved androids. Data are always expressed in percentages and arguments cumulate a crescendo of details, resulting in a seemingly unquestionable attribution of effects to causes. Even within a framework of conspiracy ideation in which the truth (at least at its general level) is known in advance, statements are supported by referring to criteria of alleged scientistic objectivism. The sources of reported knowledge are expressions of a counter-expertise that is variously legitimated. In some cases, what counts for legitimation is the experiential closeness to the reported facts (e.g. anonymous doctors sharing their personal experiences nursing sick people), which allows light to be shed on the backstage of official events. In other cases, authority comes from past or current belonging to scientific expert systems (e.g. holding one or more PhDs or working for research centres with international standing) with various, and not always clarified, paths of dissociation.

(Murru 2022)

While spreading false information about the high presence of vaccinated individuals among those who have become infected (claimed to be 'up to 90%'), websites like *Attivismo.info* attacked the Green Pass as proof that the government was defending the pharmaceutical industry and not the people (Lazzaretti 2021), given that they consider the virus to be benign and the vaccine to be dangerous ('Five doses are already in the pipeline, we will reach 17 billion euros in costs and personnel'). In the same direction, fake news was spread on the *SiAmo* blog, which forms part of the *Fronte del Dissenso*. Led by a doctor who was suspended for his anti-vaccination positions and the promotion of 'freedom of treatment', the blog attacks global finance as depriving the state of national sovereignty, and calls on people to return their membership cards to their trade unions ('It is only to preserve your privileges that you have come to terms on the worst atrocities. This is why we do not recognize you and we disown your alleged ideological clarity. You are conservatives, but today your king is naked and it was we who stripped him' (Gioia 2021).

Yet, there was little success in the attempts made to provide online space for the convergence of various groups by the so-called *Commissione Dubbio e Precauzione*, promoted by the lawyer and university professor Ugo Mattei and others (including the philosopher Giorgio Agamben), which claimed that we were in the presence of an authoritarian turn. On its website, the argument regarding the ineffectiveness of the vaccine is referred to in coarsely aggressive tones in comments such as the following:

We are furious! It was practically impossible to imagine that anyone, even political criminals, would think of requiring 'vaccine doses' for basic rights such as taking a tram, a metro, a bus, traveling by train, plane or ship, staying in hotels or B&Bs, sitting outside bars and restaurants! But that these 'measures' (which are more crazy than totalitarian!) were accepted and indeed loudly requested by the masses of zombified and howling Italiots in search of 'anti-vaxxers' … well, it is still hard to believe! The 'ease' with which we have fallen into this dystopian 'health nightmare' due to a very serious lack of genuine 'democratic antibodies' is astounding![12]

These conspiracy beliefs were subsequently spread further via comments by (mainly anonymous) participants who propose rather extreme visions of the presence of a dictatorial regime. For instance, again on the website of the *Commissione Dubbio and Precauzione,* one user commented:

The authoritarian drift of this executive, imposed on the citizens, is now clear. Parliament is deprived of its authority, the opposition is a fig leaf, politics is totally absent. The so-called scientists are committed to supporting government choices that have nothing to do with science, not to mention medicine, in a sort of scientific delirium. Almost all of the news media aggressively spread propaganda in favour of the government narrative. Medicine has been reduced to the mere propaganda of experimental drugs presented as the only, one-size-fits-all solution. Doctors no longer cure, instead they administer compounds created in computer simulations by biochemical and genetic engineers. Almost all of the judiciary does not intervene or only intervenes to give a semblance of legitimacy.

(Dipartimento Giuridico Generazioni Future 2021)

In various ways, fear is also expressed for what commentators refer to as a 'Chinese solution' which they see as the prelude to a 'chinesization' [*sic*] of society. On the same website, under the '*Nota del 2 gennaio 2022. Sul dovere di difendere lo stato costituzionale*' (Dipartimento Giuridico Generazioni Future 2022), another commentator stated that 'it is clear that the violent imposition of the GP [Green Pass] is completely unrelated to health concerns: the goal is to Chineseize [*sic*] society, assigning each individual a code of access to all human activities and to establish a system of social credits to be used to exercise one's rights'.

Declaring the lack of efficacy of the vaccines is a precondition for the claim that those who refuse vaccination are the victims of arbitrary discrimination. This can be seen, for example, in the conference organized by the *Commissione Dubbio and Prevenzione* in December 2021, at which fifty-eight activists spoke. In several speeches vaccines were defined as experimental serums that must be avoided as they were dangerous and useless, while infection was

---

[12] https://www.conoscenzealconfine.it/oms-nel-2023-guerra-ai-non-vaccinati-definiti-assassini/

presented as the preferred alternative to induce immunity. In the case of infection, a number of speakers advertised a product commonly used against parasitic worms in animals as an effective medicine. In other speeches, governments were accused of genocide and there were calls to leave the European Union, which was equated with the Soviet Union. One speaker stated that 'the pharmaceutical industry was going through an ever-deeper crisis, to save itself it was necessary to create a global pandemic and kill many people'. Compulsory vaccination is thus linked to the desire of high finance to accelerate the shift towards the digital euro and a world currency. The leader of the group, the lawyer and university professor Ugo Mattei, explained that he had decided not to get vaccinated, as, 'For once I want to see the world from the point of view of the losers of the social process. This way, I will be able to understand what it means to be excluded and I will be able to imagine a different political path' (Open 2021b).

In summary, while the number of social channels devoted to the spreading of anti-vax conspiracies was high, the connection among them mainly involved the reposting of each other's content without, however, the capacity to build sustained ties.

Expanding the comparison: The anti-vax net in Germany and Greece

A comparison with the German and the Greek case reveals many similarities in the milieus involved in the protests, albeit with different mobilizing resources in terms of pre-existing networks at the domestic level. Overall, also in these contexts, various anti-vax groups relied upon a crowdsourced organizational model, which was much more embedded in an organizational network in Germany than in Greece.

In Germany, the protests included a mix of the New Age milieu and far-right activists, with some regional differences and an evolution towards a dominance of the Far Right, which was particularly visible in the eastern regions of the country. While in the south-west of Germany, the anti-vax movement, from 2020 onwards, built upon the traditional presence of an anthroposophical network of associations and business firms, especially in the area of food, health and education (Frei and Nachtwey 2021), in the east it emerged as more influenced by the main far-right party, the AfD. In terms of an internet presence, the German anti-vax resources in 2021 included fifty-two telegram chats, forty-three Instagram and thirty-four Facebook accounts, plus thirty-five Twitter accounts, all linked together on one YouTube channel (Kleffner and Meisner 2021: 201–3). The very names of these groups (such as Doctors for the Enlightenment or Christians for the Enlightenment) refer to the right to information; however, they were involved in promoting fake news.

Just as has been observed in the Italian case study, the organizational structure in Germany developed around a crowdsourced model. Initially, the protests were promoted online by small nets of exoteric groupings, which originated in the southern states of the country. One of the earliest promoters in the New Age area was Michael Ballweg, the manager of a software firm who founded the *Querdenken 711-Initiative*, later acquiring the copyright for the *Querdenken* label. Aside from propaganda, the merchandizing of products bearing the initiative's logo spread through an intense use of social media outlets such as Telegram, YouTube and Facebook (Frei and Nachtwey 2021). Elsewhere in this area, a party named *Widerstand 2020* was founded, from which a further two splinter groups emerged, *Wir 2020* and *die Basis*, the latter of which achieved 0.99% of the vote in the state elections in Baden-Württemberg in 2021. Social media was strategically used for campaigning. This was particularly the case of Telegram, where 'ideological focal points become visible and formative, the participants find social and political confirmation and self-efficacy, where relationships, bonds and structures emerge and consolidate' (Richter et al. 2021: 76; see also Holzer 2021). This area maintained a constant presence in the German anti-vax protests, with some promoters openly endorsing QAnon conspiracies and moving towards a broad acceptance of an alliance with the Far Right.

Even more so than has been observed in Italy, the Far Right was deeply rooted in the anti-vax protest milieu, providing important organizational resources. As mentioned (see chapter 2), from the beginning of the protests, there was a particularly visible involvement of the main far-right party, the AfD, which also provided a channel of representation for anti-vax claims within both the federal and several state parliaments. Up to 40 AfD *Bundestagsabgeordnete* participated in one of the largest events in Berlin, on 29 August 2020. Moreover, there was a very visible presence of other far-right groups in the national demonstrations in Berlin in August 2020, especially the *Reichsbürger*innen*, who organized the '*Sturm auf den Reichstag*'. In the east, the Far Right was a primary organizer of anti-vax protests. However, far-right activists also had a significant presence in western states, where they called for protests and published videos on far-right media portals such as Patriots on Tour, German Defence 24 and Protest Media. In Düsseldorf, for instance, events were called by far-right groups such as the AfD, *Die Republikaner, Reichsbürger, Identitären Bewegung, Pegida NRW, Mönchengladbach* *steht auf*, *Bruderschaft Deutschland* and the *Steeler Jungs Essen*, which recruits members from right-wing hooligans (Virchow and Häusler 2020). The anti-vax network included groups promoting exclusive forms of nationalism. Throughout the country, ultra-nationalist narratives were reported on the KenFm internet channel, which included revisionist historical theses on the role of Germany in the Second World War and its supposed lack of sovereignty (Hanloser 2021).

The Far Right viewed the anti-vax protests from an instrumental perspective, as it aimed to penetrate into new constituencies. Thus, in May 2020, the neo-Nazi party *Die Rechte* published a 'Call to all nationalists' to support the 'protests of the people against the Covid dictatorship!' (cited in Virchow and Häusler 2020: 21). It presented anti-vaxxers as 'A fermented bunch in which not all, but many demonstrators are open to nationalist positions. We must seize this opportunity and not only accompany the protests as onlookers, but also set our own accents and content. ... In the middle of it instead of just being there—actively shaping the Corona protests!' (Virchow and Häusler 2020). The *Identitären Bewegung* (Identitarian movement) also called for the development of 'patriotic camps', asking 'every patriot to temporarily participate in broad alliances of convenience against the virus dictatorship and to accept compromises' (Sellner 2020). Although they did not often adhere to it, the other anti-vax groups did not distance themselves from the Far Right, instead calling for the 'old-fashioned' categories of Left and Right to be overcome. Indeed, following 29 August 2020, when many right-wing radicals appeared at the second national Coronavirus demonstration in Berlin, there was no condemnation of the Far Right by other anti-vax protestors.

The various groupings that mobilized in anti-vax protests in Greece were also similarly steered by a crowdsourced organizational model (Christou 2022), although they remained far smaller and disconnected than in the German case. In the country, an ultra-nationalist milieu had developed around the neo-Nazi Golden Dawn party, which had been the third largest party in the 2012 parliamentary elections, but was subsequently declared to be a criminal organization and dissolved. In the same milieu, the Indigenous Greek Natives (*Ellines Aftochthones Ithagenis*) and the Custodians of the Constitution (*Thematofilakes tou Sintagmatos*) spread anti-vax positions. The former operated a Facebook account and a website, which have been investigated by the Athens' Prosecutor's Office for spreading fake news and for inciting disobedience against Covid-19 related measures. The group presented itself as defender of the country that is described as having been 'sold-off' by its politicians (ibid.). The group has close links with the Greek Assembly party, which is sponsored by Artemis Sorras, an oligarch who was charged for tax evasion, the spreading of fake news and misinformation and was sentenced to three years in prison for fraud to the detriment of the financial interests of the state. Similar anti-vax positions were claimed by the Custodians of the Constitution, who present themselves as patriots, employ characteristic militaristic outfits and vehicles and often pose holding guns.

One element on the Right that is particular to the Greek context when compared with Germany is the anti-vax milieu that developed around the Greek Christian Orthodox church. As has been noted, during the pandemic, 'In most churches, Communion continued to be received by hundreds of people, all sipping from the same chalice, as is customary. The Holy Synod insisted that Communion "certainly cannot become a vector in the transmission of diseases" and that it is a "mighty manifestation of love"' (FES 2021: 6). While they initially opposed the anti-contagion measures that affected religious services and encouraged churchgoers to trust in God's protection against the virus, the Church hierarchy later softened its criticism of government measures.

Anti-vax protests in Greece also found support in a New Age milieu that had previously emerged around conspiracy ideas with weak ideological coherence, although to a far lesser extent than in the German case. This was particularly true of the supporters of the chemical trail conspiracy, which had spread during the austerity period. It claimed that unspecified evil forces had organized for poisonous substances to be sprayed from the air that would make people feel tired and passive, thus stymieing resistance against austerity measures and their consequences. Conspiracies were endorsed by a number of individual politicians, although they did not spread through the environmental social movement. The rejection of state intervention also developed in the (Anarchist) autonomist milieu, where small groups opposed anti-contagion measures as instruments of control. Among these, the Initiative against the Health Apartheid, which formed at the end of 2021, called for protests against certain Covid-19 measures. As Stella Christou (2022) has noted, 'the group stands against compulsory vaccination as an unprecedented violation of human rights, and against vaccination certificates. Certificates of vaccination are framed as "certificates of health convictions", a heuristic device that links the Green Pass with the certificate of social convictions historically issued by the Greek state confirming that the citizen was not a communist'. Taking inspiration from the Foucauldian critique of biopolitics promoted by the Italian philosopher and anti-vax activist Giorgio Agamben, the group also aimed to recruit non-vaccinated workers in the healthcare and education sectors, as well as in the police and the army. Following the introduction of compulsory vaccination for certain categories of workers and citizens over the age of 60, in the summer of 2021, the groups increased their appeals to the non-vaccinated workers in these sectors.

While in both countries the organizational structures of the anti-vax protests remained mainly local, Germany is an example of a large capacity of mobilization linked to the presence of both the support of the main far-right party and the rootedness of a commercialized and individualized New Age milieu, which focused on very individualistic visions. On the contrary, in Greece, the repression of the Far Right and the weakness of this type of New Age milieu made for a very low mobilizing capacity.

Conclusion

The anti-vax protests have been seen as a return to early-modern, rather spontaneous repertoires of action. Indeed, they have been portrayed as 'lowly organized forms of protest, with sudden gatherings of people, limited organizational structures, lack of representatives and multiplicity of protest claims. They correspond to a form of protest action that has long problematically been considered as "pre-modern" or akin to "primitive rebellion" but in fact has never disappeared from the public sphere, even in the most supposedly pacified and modernized countries' (Gerbaudo 2020: 72). Spontaneity is also emphasized in the presentation of many groups together with a sort of fluidity in the interactions between the various streams of mobilizations, especially in the earliest phases of the protests. The organizational structure of the anti-vax protests emerges, therefore, as quite localized, with a proliferation of small groups, which mainly developed online.

However, rather than 'pre-modern', the organizational model resembled the crowdsourced forms of connective action that Bennet and Segerberg (2013) have related to high connectivity and individualistic values. This can be seen in the fact that social media were used to provide toolkits for protests and other activities within the promotion of individualized forms of participation. In Italy, groups with a high presence of lawyers and health professionals specialized in offering legal and medical tools, while specific union-like groups offered support to suspended workers in the sanitary as well as the educational sectors and media outlets spread fake news. In this sense, there was not only a commercialization but also a (sort of) professionalization of the emerging groups, which aimed at stimulating self-organization.

The new groupings networked with pre-existing ones that had mobilized in previous waves of anti-vax protests as well as in anti-EU campaigns. Among the organizations that remobilized during the Covid-19 pandemic there were groups and nets that had been founded during previous waves of protest against compulsory vaccination (in particular against compulsory vaccination for children in 2017), developing structures such as homeschooling and initiatives for alternative cures and lifestyles, which had become increasingly commercialized around elitist visions based on alternative paths of consumption. Both individualism and narcissism have been nurtured in this milieu. In previous anti-vax campaigns, this milieu had encountered conservative fundamentalist groups, who opposed vaccination on the basis of religious beliefs (particularly influenced by fake news stories about the presence of human foetuses in vaccines) and the rejection of state intervention in the private sphere. Also in previous campaigns, especially those against so-called gender rights, the ultra-conservative milieu had networked with far-right groups, which often provided organizational skills. Splinter groups also aligned around anti-EU frames, claiming that they were fighting 'globalism' and defending national sovereignty. In this environment, (aspiring) movement parties focused on pandemic-related claims that they bridged with vague appeals to a 'humanistic' society and/or to a return to national sovereignty.

Given the lack of embeddedness in a resilient network, the characteristic organizational model for the mobilization of the anti-vax protests is what I would define as *disembedded crowdsourcing*. From parties to union-like groups and protest coordination committees, the shared organizational strategies are based on the creation of platforms on which instruments for mobilization are shared, in the form of documents that can be used to launch legal actions, alternative medical treatments to use in the event of contracting Covid-19, or leaflets that can be distributed locally. In this sense, the liquid structure, comprising of loose nets, primarily provided connection online without, however, being deeply rooted in real connections. While some new organizations emerged aimed at coordinating the protests, they tended to be unstable. Moreover, none of the previously existing organizations that remobilized were able to play a leading role, as fragmentation characterized the Far Right, including the neoconservative Catholic fundamentalist groups, and the New Age milieu.

The comparison with Germany and Greece has shown that, while the potential for coalition-building was limited in both countries, in Germany, the involvement of both the main far-right party and a component of a widespread anthroposophical milieu in the anti-vax protests provided for much higher mobilizing capacity than in Greece, where those conditions did not apply.

4

Framing the Anti-vax Protests

Conspiracy Beliefs in Action

The framing of protests against anti-contagion measures and vaccination during the Covid-19 pandemic: An introduction

> It depends on you, especially on the unvaccinated, who one day will be able to save humanity. Only the unvaccinated will be able to save the vaccinated who, in any case, will be forced to contact medical centres to be saved. ... I repeat: it is the unvaccinated who will be able to save humanity ... It is necessary to carefully monitor the evolution of the clinical situation, especially in vaccinated people with one, two or three doses, because there are scientific studies that have identified serious brain diseases. And we need to remove the fog that has enveloped the scientific news. Especially for people who have other pathologies, such as cancer for example, it is very important that they are not vaccinated, because there is an aluminium that enters the cells which is very carcinogenic, ... and therefore instead of treating the sick it causes them to die even sooner. Man will win if he focuses on the law of nature and only on that.
>
> **(Becchi 2022)**

This statement is part of the catastrophic vision that the (already much discussed) former Nobel Prize winner Luc Montagnier laid out. Mentioning the 'law of nature', he affirmed that humanity will only be saved by the unvaccinated. In the framing of the anti-vax protests, the reference to fake news and conspiracy theories heavily influences the narratives and symbols pitting the vaccine and vaccination as 'the evil' against the non-vaccinated as 'the good'.

Social movement studies have long considered framing processes as one of the most important aspects of mobilization. In order for a grievance to emerge, a specific strain must be cognitively linked to criticism of the ways in which authorities treat social problems. While grievances originate in material conditions, such as feelings of dissatisfaction, resentment, or indignation, the decision to mobilize on those grievances requires comparison with others and cognitive processes that produce assessments of procedural injustice (Snow 2013). In general, the responsibility for the unpleasant situation must be attributed to a deliberate producer (Klandermans 2013). Framing is all the more relevant in situations of high uncertainty when there is therefore a need to find explanations for unknown situations. In this direction, quotidian disruption acts as a dislocation that disrupts or threatens routines that individuals had previously taken for granted (Snow et al. 1998). Frames are defined as the dominant world views that guide the behaviour of social movement groups. In order to convince individuals to act, frames 'must generalize a certain problem or controversy, showing the connections with other events or with the condition of other social groups; and also demonstrate the relevance of a given problem to individual life experiences. Along with the critique of dominant representations of order and of social patterns, interpretative frames must therefore produce new definitions of the foundations of collective solidarity, transforming actors' identity in a way which favours action' (della Porta and Diani 2020: 78–9). Frames have been considered the instrumental dimension of the symbolic construction of reality by collective entrepreneurs and are very often strategically produced by the organizational leadership of a movement (Snow and Benford 1988). In William Gamson's influential work, injustice frames have been singled out as producing moral shocks that mobilize individuals into partaking in collective action (2013; also Gamson, Fireman, and Rytina 1982).

Looking more broadly at the ways in which the social reality is constructed in order to mobilize grievances into action, Snow and Benford (Snow and Benford 1988) have distinguished specific sets of frames, namely; *diagnostic* frames, which define the causes for a problematic situation; *prognostic* frames, which single out possible solutions; and *motivational* frames, which point to the motives and incentives needed for mobilization. In this sense, frame analysis has addressed the process of attribution of meaning, which lies behind any conflict through: (a) the recognition of certain occurrences as social problems; (b) the identification of possible strategies to resolve these problems; and (c) the development of motivations for acting on this knowledge. In what follows, building upon previous research (Caiani, della Porta, and Wagemann 2012), the diagnostic and prognostic levels of mobilized anti-vax groups will be analysed, distinguishing a definition of the self, which is often linked to motivational frames, and a definition of opponents, who are the 'others' against which the mobilization is oriented. This 'us' and 'them' opposition emerges as particularly relevant in the initial phases of the development of social movements, as it is linked to the very definition of the collective identity (Tilly 2003; Caiani, della Porta, and Wagemann 2012). As will be outlined in this chapter, conspiracy beliefs can affect all the different elements of the framing processes, making it possible to bridge a heterogeneous constituency. Generally speaking, in social movement studies, the framing of new events is considered to be, at least in part, path dependent on previous discursive repertoires developed within a social movement family (della Porta and Rucht 1995).

While innovating at the margins, framing processes are constrained by the subcultures that are mobilized during a wave of protest. Frame alignment broadly relies on a dynamic relationship between the development of a movement and the cultural heritage of the context in which it operates. An important form of frame alignment is frame extension, which embeds the specific concerns of a movement in more general societal goals (Snow et al. 1986), articulating the connection between a specific cause and the broad range of problems it generates. In general, emerging movements rely on the traditional heritage of social movements in a given country, although they re-elaborate them in new ways. However, reference to the past can represent an obstacle, as long-established ways of thinking and value systems can noticeably reduce the range of options available to the actor (Johnston and Klandermans 1995; Lofland 1995). If there is too strong an emphasis on tradition, frame alignment can be made particularly difficult; conversely, too weak a connection with the past reduces the capacity of the frame to spread among potential sympathizers. Importantly, it must be noted that, in 'the absence of references to one's own history and to the particular nature of one's roots, an appeal to something new risks seeming inconsistent and, in the end, lacking in legitimacy' (della Porta and Diani 2020: 86). During cycles of protest, activists aim at bridging frames which are resonant for different constituencies.

As will be seen in what follows, the protest framing in anti-vax mobilizations increasingly focused on extreme forms of individualism blended with conspiracy beliefs, in an attempt to adapt to the quickly changing pandemic scenarios (anti-lockdown, anti-mask, anti-swabs, anti-vaccine). The calls for unconstrained freedom and conspiracy beliefs that melded anti-vax narratives (including conspiracies around 5G and so-called chemtrails), ultraconservative religious views and QAnon fake news formed the basis for the encounters between the New Age and the radical Right milieus.

As noted above, there has in fact been a significant spread of conspiracy theories in the recent anti-vaccination campaigns (see also Chapter 1). From a general perspective, psychological analyses have pointed to a cognitive closure and conspiratorial mentality present in anti-vax campaigns that preceded the protests on measures aimed at controlling Covid-19. Populism has been associated with anti-vax protests as the basis of widespread mistrust, the rejection of expert knowledge, and the search for simplistic answers to complex issues, especially among those who feel 'left behind'. During the Covid-19 pandemic, the fear of an unknown challenge helped the spreading of a conspiracy mentality.

Social science research on the anti-vax protests has pointed to two main groups of mobilized actors: a New Age milieu, which has resulted in a focus on individual freedoms and alternative health practices, as well as the strategic use of the protests by the radical Right, who employ exclusionary forms of nationalism. In addition to this, a number of very small libertarian groups have attempted to connect the pandemic to developments within capitalism. Conspiracy theories have been considered to be quite rooted in these milieus and thus constitute a sort of common denominator. Within the New Age milieu, it can be observed that mistrust towards conventional medicine interacts with an increase in individualistic narratives. Conspiracies, including those on 5G, chemtrails, and vaccination in general, had penetrated the New Age milieu already before the pandemic. In the Far Right, during the backlash new forms of exclusive nationalism have been connected with neoconservative religious values and anti-EU narratives. Far-right groups, which have often provided important resources for anti-vax protests, have regularly been found to support conspiracy theories. In most cases these theories are aimed at linking the spread of Covid-19 to immigration, especially 'illegal' immigration, as well as to ethnic minorities. The tendency to believe superstitious and exoteric statements (which is particularly widespread among right-wing voters) is fuelled by 'a narrative that binds fear, excessive demands and powerlessness and gives space to the (regressive) desire to live in a world perceived as controllable or a reconciled (primordial) state with nature' (Schließler, Hellweg, and Decker 2020: 295).

The analysis of the framing processes in the Italian anti-vax campaigns presented below identifies the diagnostic frame in the expansion of the powers of a (hidden) elite through various global plots aimed at exercising total control over citizens. The prognostic solution is the defence of (assumed) previously existing liberties, primarily related with freedom, defined in a negative sense as the primacy of individual choice over the collective good. Oppositional frames targeted what was seen as a large global conspiracy, carried out by politicians, corporations, and Big Pharma, which aimed at establishing a sanitary dictatorship. The identity framing involved a call for individual freedoms, which were considered as being jeopardized by an international elite of politicians, scientists, and journalists with the intention of imposing a global order, pointing to the resistance of a persecuted population of enlightened and critical individuals fighting for their individual freedoms against a powerful global elite, supported by loyal serfs (such as journalists and experts) and a mass of vaccinated 'zombies'. Thus, different strands present at the beginning of the mobilization tend to be bridged in action through the diffusion of conspiratorial views. As framing is linked to organizational networks and political opportunities, the specific mix of the main components may vary in space and time. The presentation of the Italian case study will be followed by a comparison with the German and Greek cases, which will confirm the presence of similar frames in the various contexts, albeit with certain levels of adaptation to the discursive opportunities in the latter two countries. In the conclusion, some of the implications of the use of conspiracy beliefs for the effects of the framing processes will be outlined.

Diagnostic frames: The sanitary dictatorship

Two main sets of diagnostic frames addressed the presumed health and socio-political consequences of Covid-19. While the former were mainly cited by organizations concerned with New Age visions and the latter by those more oriented towards (right-wing) politics, these were commonly combined, with a discursive radicalization taking place on both sides around conspiracy narratives.

  While the groups diverge on the degree to which the very existence of the pandemic was denied, there was considerable convergence in framing Covid-19 as 'just a flu', that is, an easily cured disease characterized by low levels (or at least declining levels) of lethality. The numbers of deaths caused by Covid-19 were consequently considered to be exaggerated (given the widespread use of tests or the specific criteria for counting cases, which sometimes included those who happened to have the disease when they died of other illnesses rather than only those who died specifically due to the virus). The deaths were, moreover, often attributed to the use of paracetamol in the treatment of patients or the vaccination itself. Test swabs were also considered to be unreliable or even risky, and it was argued that their use, seen as promoted by the pharmaceutical industry and political elites, was aimed at increasing the perception of a spread of the contagion, imposing costs on the state and on individuals (this was especially the case for PCR tests, which were claimed by anti-vax activists to provide false positives 'in 90% of cases').

In addition to the denial of the severity of the disease, there was a specific attack on vaccines as being an (American) form of 'gene therapy'. This criticism of vaccination builds on previously existing arguments on vaccines more generally, albeit with a particular stress on the specific nature of the vaccines used in targeting the Covid-19 virus. As part of this narrative, vaccines are defined as ineffective in both the short and the long term, as it is claimed in anti-vaccination statements that not only do they not prevent contagion, but that they do not even reduce hospitalization numbers or deaths. Claims that there is a lack of scientific evidence on the efficacy of vaccination are bridged with statements about the risks that it poses, including myocardial and pericardial diseases, compromised fertility, various types of cancer, paralysis of the immune system, poisoning related to the protein spike used in the vaccines, and the spread of more dangerous variants of the virus that are resistant to vaccines. A specific element in the criticisms of the Covid-19 vaccines revolves around claims of DNA manipulation, along with claims that 'chimpanzee adenovirus' or human foetuses have been injected into the bodies of vaccinated individuals. In a larger sense, this is linked to what is considered to be a mass experiment, as the anti-vaxxers assert that Covid vaccines had only received emergency authorization, without going through the normal monitoring procedures to ensure the safety of the treatment. While some groups are open to the selective vaccination of specific categories of individuals, those who had previously been active against the vaccination of children and the elderly consider any vaccine as dangerous due to their supposed long-term consequences, use of which by children they link to autism; and by the elderly, to reduced life expectancy. Of particular note is the fact that in some narratives, vaccination is presented as a point of no return, with a dark fate predicted for the '*sierati*' (i.e. those who have been administered the 'serum').

All of these claims converge in a meta frame that presents the refusal to be vaccinated as an expression of 'individual freedom from vaccination'. The arguments against compulsory vaccination point to the specific characteristics of the existing vaccines in terms of what is argued is their lack of capacity in preventing contagion as well as the novelty of the use of a genetic treatment that renders both their effectiveness and effects uncertain. Thus, a document produced by the *Movimento 3V* puts forward 'The 17 reasons given by doctors and scientists that convince us not to get vaccinated against Covid-19' (Gruppo Salute 2020):

1. Because I'm not a guinea pig 2. Because I could still get sick 3. Because I could still infect others. 4. Because I could spread more dangerous variants of the virus

5. Because no real virus statistics are known, only those based on unreliable swabs 6. Because there are effective cures for Covid 7. Because I carry out primary prevention 8. Because the medium and long-term side effects of the vaccine are not known 9. Because the side effects could include death 10. Because the Spike protein causes strokes and thrombosis 11. Because my fertility could be compromised 12. Because the pharmaceutical companies take no responsibility 13. Because no mRNA drug has ever been used in the world before 14. Because I refuse to inject foreign DNA into my body 15. Because in Italy there is no active pharmacovigilance in general 16. Because without knowing it I might already be immune 17. Because I have not received the legally necessary information to make a choice.

As an expression of the New Age wing of the anti-vax campaign, the *Movimento 3V* promotes itself as 'the only party that demands truth and puts the well-being and health of the human beings at the center of all political action'.[1] With a strong focus of health issues, their program calls for the abolition of all anti-contagion measures and freedom of therapeutic choice (with blind faith in 'homeopathic medicine') including:

1.General rejection of the measures adopted at a national and regional level for the alleged containment of the spread of Covid-19, which have proved to be contradictory, disproportionate to the health risk, scientifically and medically inconsistent or incorrect and causing enormous damage in terms of primary prevention, the possibilities of economic sustenance and the psychophysical equilibrium of the population, areas with a direct impact on the health of the citizens. 2. Fight against social distancing, Compulsory Health Treatments, care or diagnosis obligations and invasive health devices. 3. Fight against vaccination passport and DNA profiling projects. 4. Opposition to any provision that prevents, in particular in the medical/scientific field, the safeguarding of the principle of truth, communication and integration of knowledge. 5. Opposition to any vaccination obligation currently existing and its effects on the health, the families and social conditions of citizens, including the obligations for professional and sporting purposes envisaged for personnel of the security forces, the armed forces, for school operators, health workers and athletes.

The dangerous effects of the 'serum' in destroying the 'natural' DNA of individuals are often pointed to. One of the most extreme, but often cited, representations of the supposed risks of the Covid-19 vaccine was presented

---

[1] https://www.movimento3v.it/.

in a speech at a demonstration in Milan on 15 January 2022 by the anti-vax icon, Nobel Prize winner Luc Montagnier, who was cited as claiming:

> The protein that was used in the vaccines for this virus is actually toxic and a poison. … There have been many deaths, even young sportsmen who have had major problems due to this vaccine. It is an absolute crime to give these vaccines to children today. Let's stop mass vaccination. It can also cause very serious nerve diseases in the brain. Due to the long-term effects of this vaccine many people are dying.
>
> **(Becchi 2022).**

The catastrophic consequences of the 'gene serum', connected to the plots created by a 'new multinational state of the cyberpharmaceutical industries', are cited over and over again in the online chats and blogs of different types of groups. In a comment on *Replica Costruttiva e Invito al Dialogo* del *Dipartimento Giuridico di Generazioni Future* (Generazioni Future 2022b), a certain Dott. Ramingo attacks what he terms 'capitalist science', stating, 'They will not inject me with gene implants or, even worse, nanotechnology.' Fake news is also posted referring to 'the "sudden" deaths of sportsmen, actors, musicians between 20 and 50 years old all over the world which continue, [while] regime megaphones such as Yahoo News report one or two per day … with the only reason for death given as "found at home" or "sudden illness". In those who receive the various doses, cases of paralysis are multiplying, and even more so cases of "St. Anthony's fire"'. Given the presumed risks of vaccination, all measures taken with the aim of incentivizing participation in the vaccination campaign are stigmatized as arbitrary. As a result, the situation is framed as 'discrimination against the unvaccinated'. For instance, in a '*Lettera di solidarietà al personale scolastico per la sanzione della sospensione dal lavoro e dello stipendio*' (Goccia 2022), compulsory vaccination is considered as attacking both one's right to self-determination and the right to work, given the fact that 'The sanction that deprives a worker of the means of subsistence on the basis of his convictions, when it is not evident that with his resulting conduct he is causing damage to the community, we believe must be strongly rejected in principle, also for the juridical-ethical-political consequences that such a precedent can set.' Thus, vaccination is considered as a way of 'putting people to sleep' and a dangerous judicial precedent.

Deprived of its epidemiological efficacy as well as of the capacity to convince individuals of the need for vaccination (which is also claimed to be useless as there are already high rates of vaccination), the Green Pass (as a proxy for compulsory vaccination) is accused of increasing social inequality, the exploitation of women and the discrimination of foreigners (vaccinated with non-recognized vaccines), reducing sociability for the young, and producing environmental pollution. The Green Pass is also accused of denying inalienable rights, through what is portrayed as its attacks on privacy. In this sense, it is claimed that measures on compulsory vaccination turn individuals into criminals for what they are, not what they have done (just as has been the case in various countries if one were communist, gay, or Jewish). By stigmatizing groups of citizens, the argument goes, it produces second-class citizens, creating divisions in society that could be equated with apartheid, introducing a state of detention and deprivation through the discrimination of a group of individuals. Anti-contagion measures are also considered to be non-constitutional (as the decision of the Constitutional Court no. 5/2018 is said to limit compulsory vaccination to safe vaccines), with activists pointing to the disproportion between the risks and restrictions placed on freedoms.

The Green Pass (which, as mentioned, served to restrict access to certain spaces only to people who have either been vaccinated, recovered from infection, or tested negative for Covid-19) is in fact defined as an instrument of discrimination, as it is aimed at increasing vaccination numbers (or, as is commonly argued, as a surrogate for compulsory vaccination). For instance, an 'Appello al Governo per l'esenzione dal green pass per gli studenti che utilizzano mezzi di trasporto pubblici' denounces the specific discrimination of the vaccination certificate for foreigners, or those vaccinated with vaccines that have not been recognized by the EU (Goccia 2021). Thus, for instance, the requirement to show a valid Green Pass to access schools, universities, or public transport is considered to be a measure that denies the right to education for those who 'in full accordance with the law, have held off on vaccinating their children while waiting for more exhaustive scientific evidence; it is in effect a serious violation of the constitutional principle of the right to education, as it deprives unvaccinated students of the right to go to school using public transport' (ibid.). The same document considers the existing security protocols as sufficient to avoid contagion, also pointing to the specific economic discrimination related with the cost of the tests for large or poorer families or the assumed gender discrimination of the mothers that are forced to stay at home with their (unvaccinated) children, as well as at the environmental impact of the increased use of private transport.

The extreme (but very widespread) version of the discrimination frame employed defines the unvaccinated as a 'persecuted minority' in what is presented, both in text and images, as similar to the persecution of Jewish people during the Shoah (see also Chapter 2). Thus, an 'Appello dei docenti universitari: "No al green pass"', invoking Article 32 of the Italian Constitution as well as EU Regulation n.953/2021, evokes 'other historical precedents that we would never have wanted to recall', stating that 'All of us, however, consider the discrimination introduced against a minority to be unjust and illegitimate' (AttoPrimo 2021). There are accusations that 'second-class citizens' are being created, as 'the "Green Card" divides Italian society into A League citizens, who continue to enjoy their rights, and B League citizens, who instead see a restriction of those fundamental rights guaranteed to them by the Constitution (equality, personal freedom, work, study, freedom of association, freedom of movement, freedom of opinion)'.[2] Similarly, in the 'Lettera degli studenti di Bergamo contro il Green Pass' (1 September 2021), the claim is that there has been an imposition of

> a principle of discrimination, legitimized by reasons presented as medical or scientific, which appears to us to be the polar opposite of that same inclusivity etymologically established upon the foundation of the institution of the university. With this discriminative and divisive provision, all those who, through legitimate personal choice, do not intend to subject themselves to invasive health treatments and at their own expense, are in fact excluded from the right to study and from the services provided by the university—or their accessibility is severely limited.
>
> **(Studenti contro il Green Pass 2021)**

What is more, the Green Pass is considered as proof of an authoritarian turn, which it is claimed will go as far as what is framed as a 'state of exception'. The existence of a despotic regime is denounced in particular in several interventions by the philosopher Giorgio Agamben, which were circulated in various outlets. In 'Una comunità nella società', he wrote:

> Today Italy, like a political laboratory of the West in which the strategies of the dominant powers are elaborated in advance in their most extreme form, is a country in disarray both humanly and politically, in which an unscrupulous and determined tyranny has allied itself with the masses in the grip of a pseudo-religious terror, ready to sacrifice not only what were once called constitutional freedoms, but even all warmth in human relations.
>
> **(Agamben 2021c)**

In this vision, the management of the pandemic is presented as the implementation of a state of exception. During his speech at the conference on 'Le politiche pandemiche', on 10 November 2021 in Turin, Agamben once again

---

[2] https://nogreenpassdocenti.wordpress.com/ (accessed 30 October 2021).

referred to his conception of the state of exception as a situation in which 'on the one hand the law is theoretically in force, but has no force, it is not applied, and on the other, provisions and measures that do not have the force of law, acquire force', stating that, 'If then, as is happening today, the state of exception becomes the rule, the eclipse of the law is all the more visible and gives rise to the abolition of that fundamental principle of our law which is the certainty of the law.' In this 'administrative state', there is 'a generalized state of minority, which citizens who constantly have to show their Green Pass mistake instead for a guarantee of freedom, without thinking that, just as it has been granted, the authorization can be withdrawn' (Generazioni Future 2021a). Similarly, in '*La nuda vita e il vaccino*', he claims that 'the epidemic shows beyond any possible doubt that humanity no longer believes in anything except in preserving its bare existence as it is at any price. …. that is, a life that is neither properly animal nor truly human, but in which the decision between the human and the non-human takes place constantly', as had happened in the past for slaves, barbarians, or the Jews in Nazi concentration camps (Agamben 2021a).

One of the master frames that is shared by various components of the antivax movement is the definition of the measures aimed at stopping the spread of Covid-19 as proving the existence of a dictatorship. Among others, the leader of *Genova Libera Piazza*, the group that organized several protests in the Ligurian city, claimed that the vaccine was used as an instrument for the total control of the population:

We are in a full technocratic dictatorship with very clear dystopian developments, justified by an 'emergency' based on manipulated data and pseudo-scientific concepts. We are talking about a disease for which there has always been a cure, which is knowingly denied by politicians and health authorities …. The denial of the autopsies that would have revealed the exact pathology, the lack of information on the fact that the disease could be safely treated, the referral to the 'salvific' experimental 'vaccine' and the cloak of political-media terror, destroyer of the primary immune defence of the individual, which is their moral reaction, are in fact genuine 'state crimes' and systemic crimes against the much heralded 'public health'. All this, served on a plate by a global propaganda apparatus, which is essentially private, that is so powerful and elaborate that it is the envy of 'good old' Goebbels. The purpose of this global manoeuvre, which involves the destruction-reconstruction of production, economy and finance with the aim of definitively placing it in the hands of global corporations, is to subjugate every man on the face of the earth, and in fact life itself, to a total, capillary, unavoidable and definitive control and manipulation.

(Franceschini 2021b)

Somewhat paradoxically, the denunciation of a dictatorial state is also dominant in the pandemic narrative on the Far Right. *Forza Nuova*, in particular, contested the very seriousness of the virus, stressing the danger that the 'globalist' management of the pandemic posed in terms of the instauration of a 'sanitary dictatorship' by a globalist elite that is at the service of China and the WTO. The group thus launched a 'struggle of national liberation' in the name of the freedom 'to go out, to work, to meet, to play sport' and to express 'the power to decide the destiny of our people and our nation' (in Frazzetta 2022: 209). Indeed, *Forza Nuova* built its narrative of the pandemic on the conspiracy visions of a 'new world order' supported by an alliance of the WTO, pharmaceutical multinationals, and China. In this narrative, Covid-19 is considered to be nothing more than a flu, while the anti-vax positions are supported and all anti-contagion measures are seen as not only useless but also counterproductive. Thus, in challenging the 'crazy quarantine', the group states that 'it facilitates infection within the family, with increasing hospitalization and deaths' (in ibid.: 207). Inviting its followers to disobey the anti-contagion rules, *Forza Nuova* stated that 'it is a time for lions, not for rabbits' (ibid.: 211). Although *Casa Pound* considered the virus to be a real threat whose consequences were increased by the weakening of the public health system during the austerity crisis, it appealed to right-wing parties such as the Lega and Brothers of Italy to promote legislation in parliament against what League claimed was the centralization of the then Prime Minister Giuseppe Conte, who they termed a 'small dictator'. On the Far Right, the framing of the pandemic was also bridged with the appeal to regain national sovereignty and to take full control of the national economy. In this line, the EU was accused of jeopardizing the national economic interests of the country as well as repressing national cultures by supporting an invasion by foreign people and ethnic replacement (ibid.: 81–7, 105, 111).

As a consequence of these narratives, Covid-19 vaccinations are portrayed as an illegitimate compulsory sanitary treatment, which essentially sanction the end of the state of law. While emergency legislation disempowers the parliament, it is claimed that a technocratic dictatorship is aimed at bringing about a Global Reset. A primary example of this conspiracy vision can be seen in the writings of the nationalist group *Liberiamo l'Italia*, which presents 'Operation Covid' as a plot drawn up by cosmopolitan 'cybercapitalism' against national sovereignty:

> Operation Covid is used by global elites as a weapon to implement the Great Reset, or to reshape the entire social system. For many reasons, with the guilty complicity of the national ruling classes, Italy is being used by these elites as a laboratory to

implement their strategic plans for social restructuring and as a test bed to gauge the reaction of the popular masses.

(Liberiamo l'Italia 2021)

Conspiracy beliefs bridge the 'state of exception' frame with some basic anti-vax arguments. The Green Pass is depicted as useless given the fact that vaccinated individuals can spread the virus. This can be seen in a post entitled '*Bisogna difendere lo Stato costituzionale*' by the *Commissione Dubbio e Precauzione*, which notes:

> It has now also been established—disproving previous triumphalist assertions—that the vaccine only protects from infection to a limited extent (by a factor equal to about three times the risk of unvaccinated people). In the face of this evidence, the Green Pass loses any justification as a health measure: being vaccinated does not guarantee that the holder is immune or cannot infect others.

(Terra Nuova 2022)

Moreover, in a statement titled 'Sulle misure "di contenimento dell'epidemia" adottate dal Governo il 29/12/21' the *Commissione Dubbio e Precauzione* affirms that swabs are more effective than vaccines: 'In light of the factual findings that have emerged so far, it is clear that the tightening of restrictions on unvaccinated individuals has nothing to do with combating the epidemic' (Generazioni Future 2021b).

In summary, the diagnostic frame combined a scepticism towards both the seriousness of the Covid-19 virus (often defined as a flu) and, even more so, the efficacy of the vaccines with a denunciation of anti-contagion measures as attacking individual freedoms. With the passing of time, the various frames converged in a conspiracy vision of an alleged plot by a tiny cosmopolitan elite who is accused of exploiting or even having produced the virus in order to impose a dictatorial order.

Prognostic frames: Back to normality

While the statements and documents produced by groups involved in anti-vax protests afford a large amount of space to the diagnostic frames, their prognostic frames are much less developed. In fact, an explicit assumption is commonly made that mobilization must focus on the (very) minimal area of agreement shared by the different groups, i.e. a return to the *status quo ante* of assumed freedom and natural laws. This is articulated on two prognostic levels: one refers to how to address the virus and the other deals with how to fight what is considered to be an authoritarian regime.

On the medical level, prognostic frames varied between those who acknowledge the existence of Covid-19 and those who deny it. Among the former, suggestions ranged from mass covid testing and hygiene protocols (face masks, social distancing or even staying at home) to selective compulsory vaccination, the abolition of the Green Pass for young people, the end of the requirement to wear masks at schools and the promotion of more traditional vaccines (with coverage for five years). Where groups or individuals were partially in denial of the existence of the pandemic, there was a tendency to champion natural treatments and dietary solutions aimed at keeping the immune system active or even to cure the disease. Alternative treatments for Covid-19 that were advertised include ozone therapy, hydroxychloroquine, ivermectin, Vitamins C and D, dexamethasone, enoxaparin, hyperimmune plasma, and monoclonal antibodies. The use of alternative home remedies was advertised as a substitute for the 'paracetamol and watchful waiting' protocol promoted by the Italian Ministry of Public Health. Among the most extreme denialists, there were appeals to attempt to gain immunization through infection as well as calls to place vaccinated individuals in quarantine (as they are accused of producing mutations in the virus).

There was also a spread of an individualistic conception of health as related to personal choices and, therefore, responsibility. With regard to how the virus should be treated, there were calls for home remedies and the strengthening of the immune system through peculiar diets and 'alternative cures'. As is the case for many other activists, in a comment on the site of *Commissione Dubbio e Precauzione* (under the '*Nota del 2 gennaio 2022. Sul dovere di difendere lo stato costituzionale*') a user declared her fierce mistrust of 'allopathic' medicine, stating that,

> in the directives issued by the Government there has never been the slightest openness for those who have always and only taken care of themselves, and have prevented illness by using natural cures and nutrition, thus maintaining their immune defences in the best possible way. A single cure—which is a gene serum that they incorrectly call a vaccine—cannot be the solution for everyone. I have never taken allopathic medicines, why should I start taking them now? And if I have some adverse reactions—I live alone—who will cure me ???

In his reply to this post, another user reacted by suggesting isolation as a solution:

> I completely agree with you! I am also in the same situation. I have always followed precise measures to avoid getting sick, which involved a great deal of 'sacrifice' when compared to a normal life, so I have never been a burden on the health

system. And even now, as an unvaccinated person, I continue to avoid those risky contexts where I could become infected and stay at home most of the time.

(Difendersi Ora 2022)

The use of alternative cures is promoted, either directly or indirectly, on several anti-vax websites, where commercial adverts about alternative diets and natural remedies are also often published. A good example of this can be seen on the website of the *Commissione Dubbio e Precauzione* (comment on the 'Nota del 2 gennaio 2022. Sul dovere di difendere lo stato costituzionale') in relation to the supposed repression of home remedies. Calling paracetamol 'the real killer of the 2020 massacre', a commenter suggested the following:

In the first days of symptoms generic flu drugs have prevented all of the elderly people I know who used them from degenerating beyond the typical flu symptoms, and similar results have been repeatedly demonstrated, not by me but by physicians working in the field, who have also come together in organizations that have been demanding to be listened to for more than a year, having saved over 80% of their infected patients by avoiding hospitalization; if only the very deaf and bloated imperial body known as the 'Ministry of Health' had listened to them for even just 5 minutes in the months and months up to this point. … The evidence of the effectiveness [of these treatments] is clear, but its use is prohibited and those who prescribe it are even threatened with radiation for violating the 'paracetamol and watchful waiting protocol' that, lowering the fever without affecting the inflammation in the least, was and is the real cause of the majority of deaths, thanks to the anti-medical imposition by the 'Imperial Ministry'.

(Difendersi Ora 2022)

Aside from Covid-19, the prognostic faming focuses on a 'return to freedom'. In some groups, this is expressed as the promotion of a 'human society, different, happy, solid and solidary', of an ethical reform towards 'humanism', the freedom to cure oneself according to one's will and homeschooling. As with many others in the anti-vax galaxy, one of the main exponents of this position, the *Movimento 3V*, links individual 'dignity' not only to freedom but also to an individual conception of health as related to one's own choice of healthy lifestyles:

The freedom of human beings has now disappeared on the basis of hypothetical medical-scientific reasons which, according to doctors and scientists, are non-existent, false or incorrect down to their very foundations. … Human beings cannot be guinea pigs subjected to radio frequencies or drugs that are unsafe, unchecked or solely tested on humans, in the name of progress or a concept of health that is devoid of any human logic. Any obligation or pressure that affects the health of the individual in even a potentially risky way must be considered a crime against humanity ... The physical, psychological and spiritual health of the human being is guaranteed for all through healthy lifestyles, proper nutrition, an unpolluted environment and harmonious sociality.[3]

In addition to this, self-determination is promoted as the right to inviolability of the body, which is linked to the claims to reinstate the constitutional rights to education, work, movement, health, information, speech, and demonstration.

'Moving beyond Covid' is a common aim that makes it possible to find shared ground beyond the traditional Left and Right division. As such, the activist Andrea Zhok, in promoting the establishment of a new political entity, points to the need to go beyond the old divisions, stating that:

While this situation has, on the one hand, destroyed many illusions, it has also opened up an unexpected and unhoped for human dimension on the other. We have discovered ideologically transversal affinities and solidarity, we have managed to find comfort in the words and deeds of hitherto unknown people, with whom a human connection has been established based on a primary sense of freedom, respect for the individual and justice. This connection is 'pre-political', or perhaps better, it is originally political in the primitive sense of the term: it is human trust in the ability to cooperate. The definitive abandonment of the political categories of the past, starting with 'Right' and 'Left', an abandonment that has been developing for some time, has received its definitive consecration. ... as if the loss of work and the inability to access restaurants, cultural sites, etc. were not enough, European governments today are competing with each other to invent new forms of harassment against the new public enemy number 1: the unvaccinated.

(Zhok 2021c)

Anti-vax frames are also bridged with anti-EU ones, targeting a cosmopolitan elite in the name of national sovereignty. From a political perspective, one of the main claims emanating from pre-existing splinter parties, such as *Ancora Italia*, *Italexit*, *Alternativa*, or *Vox Italia* is the re-establishment of national sovereignty, which includes both monetary and alimentary sovereignty. For the group *Liberiamo l'Italia*, who aspire to become the main nucleus for an anti-vax party, the framing of the pandemic is linked to the call to 'free Italy'.

[3] https://www.movimento3v.it/visione-3v/ (accessed 30 October 2021).

This can be seen in the promotion of a demonstration on 12 October 2021, in which the group proclaimed that:

> Italy is at a turning point. Either European demands will be rejected once and for all, or the country's decline will be unstoppable. Poverty, unemployment and insecurity can and must end, but European rules prevent us from doing so. While they guarantee all rights to private and speculative finance, they prevent states from pursuing the common good. The Italian people are deprived of any rights, even the right to escape the crisis. For the EU, the only policy permitted remains that of sacrifices, while the 1948 Constitution itself is trampled on by modern day Euro-German legal and financial tanks. It is time to escape from this cage. Italy has the resources and the means to get out of the situation in which it was thrown, almost thirty years ago, by an irresponsible and corrupt political class. … Liberation is possible, but you must believe it. … Let's free Italy!
>
> **(Liberiamo l'Italia n.d.)**

The reference to the return to a pre-Covid 19 world with a defence of individual choices and the fatherland also characterized the *Fronte del Dissenso*:

> The minimum agenda consists of a project for: a) the complete restoration of the *status quo ante*, of the situation prior to the introduction of the blocks, bans, current restrictions; b) the introduction of positive norms that prevent similar degeneration in the future. On such an agenda there can be massive integral and transversal convergence … A programme and a minimum statute can be agreed without too much difficulty, in the awareness that the main mandate is defensive and restores betrayed constitutional instances.
>
> **(Fronte del Dissenso 2021)**

Indeed, the *Fronte del Dissenso* declares that it condemns 'the instrumental use of Sars CoV-2, a picklock to justify the initiation of a "creative destruction" aimed at creating an economic system of impoverishment of large masses of the population through savage competition and generating permanent austerity', adding that it 'defends the principles of the inviolability of the body and free therapeutic choice'. Rejecting 'a power that aims to destroy individuals, perhaps to deliver body and soul to the interests of multinationals', it as mentioned rejects the distinction between Left, Center and Right as an instrument of the elite oriented to divide the citizens. Instead, words and symbols appeal to 'the Fatherland', with abundant use of the green-red-white colours of the Italian flag (ibid.).

Connecting anti-EU positions with the opposition to vaccination, in November 2021, the conference of the delegates of *Liberiamo l'Italia* deliberated that 'The project of the ruling oligarchy is clear: to reshape society and individuals themselves, in order to obtain obedience, social discipline, surveillance of souls and bodies within a new totalitarian regime that is far more sophisticated than in the twentieth century.' Expanding on the need to fight against the 'Great Reset', the document singled out the movement against the Green Pass as the real opposition, lamenting, however, the presence within it of a tendency to escape the political struggle and to 'withdraw into small communities'. In this direction, the proposal is 'the unity of all the forces of constitutional sovereignty together with those that are fighting against emergencyism and for the defence of individual and collective freedoms within a federation of democratic patriotic forces aiming "to free themselves from the European cage"'.[4]

As time progressed, the framing became more and more extreme in its adoption of various types of conspiracies. Conspiracy visions of a global plot to be opposed through a return to national sovereignty are in fact presented in various media outlets. For instance, '*Effetti Avversi: raccolta di critica sulla gestione politica e sanitaria della pandemia*' published contributions by academics in the anti-vax milieu, who elaborate on the critique of pandemic policies as the product of global capitalism. This is the case of Fabio Vighi, a university professor in the UK, who, in '*Paradigma Covid: collasso sistemico e fantasma pandemico*', presents the pandemic as an invention of global capitalism:

A year and a half after the arrival of the Virus, someone may have wondered why the ruling class, unscrupulous by its nature, has put the profit machine in the freezer in the face of a pathogen that is almost exclusively raging against unproductive subjects—those over 80 who, among other things, have been putting the pension system to the test for some time. Why, suddenly, all this zeal? *Cui prodest?* Only those unfamiliar with the amazing adventures of GloboCap (global capitalism) can

---

[4] The document also notes the gap between the actual electoral results and what is considered as a potential electoral base 'estimated today at around 30%': 'While the idea of a civic opposition able to gather the best of the old M5s (see Rome) proved to be absolutely the loser, three were the most significant results: that of the list headed by Ugo Mattei in Turin (2.4 %), that of Paragone in Milan (2.9%), and that of the 3V Movement in some smaller cities (Trieste, Rimini and Ravenna), oscillating between 2.9 and 4.6%. ... We call this base "potential hard core", because on the one hand (given the absence of a sufficiently strong general identity) it is clear that we are facing a sort of "hard core", but on the other hand it is still only potential, given that only in the presence of certain conditions (media leaders already known or particular local settlement situations) did it translate into effective electoral consensus.' (ibid).

delude themselves that the system closes its doors out of charitable spirit. The great predators of oil, weapons, and vaccines don't give a damn about humanity.

(Vighi 2021)

A similar tone is set by the right-wing nationalist group *Ancora Italia* in a manifesto published on its website. Attacking the Green Pass and compulsory vaccination, the group demands 'sovereignty: not only that of the State, but also—let us not forget—the mental sovereignty of the community individual, first and foremost; that is, the ability to gain immunity from the herd and to resist the single, politically correct and ethical mindset' (Ancora Italia Palermo n.d.).

A common thread in these narratives is the idea of an emergency to be addressed through a new constitutional phase, with some calls for the participation of citizens and a generic appeal to politics. The call is therefore to 'structure the resistance to the Regime in the medium term … in all aspects of life but at the same time working on overturning it and therefore building that process of liberation from the Regime and conquest of the State now held by the officials of the Regime' (Studenti contro il Green Pass 2022b). In the '*Manifesto per la dichiarazione di emergenza giuridica*', the *Commissione Dubbio e Precauzione* similarly calls for the forging of a new constitution, as they claim that, 'We are facing a national legal emergency and this, like the others, must be declared, and here it is declared! … On 9 March 2020 the state of law was abolished by renouncing the tripartition of power' (Generazioni Future 2022a).

However, in spite of somewhat shared visions on the above, when it comes to prognostic frames, major tensions emerge within the archipelago of anti-vax protestors. According to one activist, among the array of anti-vax groups it is possible to single out a number of trends:

(1) that of democratic republicanism, which also includes socialist and anarchist currents; (2) that of traditionalist Catholicism, within which one finds the reactionary component … and also certain fascist groupings; (3) the liberal trend, within which there are both genuine anarcho-liberals and liberalists; (4) the phantasmagorical grouping, which also includes generic new age spiritualism, for whom Gandhism undoubtedly provides a core political figure; (5) what we could define as communitarian groups—in this case linked by the idea of 'founding, here and now, alternative communities of life outside the systemic perimeter, based on strong ethical and value constraints'.

(Pasquinelli 2021)

It is perhaps unsurprising, then, that internal conflicts emerge between those who propose a political path, including participation in elections, and those who would prefer instead to retreat into small communities. This is especially the case as mobilization begins to decline. The more isolated the anti-vaxxers feel, the more widespread the appeals to build secluded societies. Resistance through retreat into a sort of clandestine life, based on self-organized communities, is particularly propounded by the philosopher George Agamben:

> In these conditions, without abandoning every possible instrument of immediate resistance, dissidents need to think about creating something like a society within society, a community of friends and neighbours within the society of enmity and distance. The form of this new clandestine reality, which will have to make itself as autonomous from the institutions as possible, will be meditated and tested from time to time, but only they will be able to guarantee human survival in a world that has more or less devoted itself to conscious self-destruction.
>
> (Agamben 2021c)

Although the political trend within anti-vax protesters condemned such communitarianism as nihilistic, it was itself divided by bitter competition for a supposed electoral base that failed to materialize. Thus, one activist noted:

> if you pay due attention to the debate within the communitarian component of the anti-Green Pass movement, if you analyse the ideas in circulation with the necessary scruples, you will discover not only a great deal of naïve abstractness, but you will also come across theoretical carelessness and real abstruseness ... we do not believe that catastrophe is inevitable; we believe that there are still the space, time and conditions to prevent the advent of what we have termed cybercapitalism. If we are right, no self-exclusion from the world is permitted, no escape from the political struggle is acceptable. If we are right, we cannot escape the POLITICAL duty of consolidating the Resistance, of structuring it as a hegemonic and constituent popular counter-power.
>
> (Pasquinelli 2021)

In summarizing the above, it can be said that the prognostic framing called for the abolition of anti-contagion measures in the name of the defence of individual freedoms, with proposals to address the virus through alternative lifestyles, natural treatments, or even voluntary infection. As the pandemic progressed, conspiratorial thinking pushed for a convergence on the call to resist the alleged dictatorship with shared appeals to re-establishing the 'natural order'.

Identity frames: A heroic minority

A third element that is closely linked to the diagnostic and prognostic frames is the definition of the identity of the mobilizing groups. Social movement studies have often addressed the cognitive and affective mechanisms related with the transformation of stigmatized identities into valuable ones (della Porta and Diani 2020: Chapter 4). In fact, identity framing is aimed at motivating action, and as such, catalysing the mobilization of the claimed constituency. This task is particularly important for a movement of individuals who present themselves as an 'oppressed minority'.

There are two main sets of identity frames in the anti-vax narrative in Italy, one which points to those opposing vaccination and the Green Pass as 'poor victims' and another which presents them as 'resisting heroes'. In considering themselves as victims (just as Jewish people or slaves in the past), anti-vaxxers often use language that laments their stigmatization as the excluded, the powerless, the 'poor devils sent to the slaughter', second-class citizens, or even the victims of a social experiment. Thus, commonly used symbols include the yellow star that Jewish people were forced to wear during the Nazi regime in Germany or the striped vests given to prisoners in the extermination camps during the Holocaust (see Chapter 2). Along these lines, in an intervention titled '*Cittadini di seconda classe*', Agamben noted: 'As happens every time a despotic emergency regime is established and constitutional guarantees are suspended, the result is, as happened for the Jews under fascism, the discrimination of a category of men, who automatically become second class citizens' (Agamben 2021b).

Anti-vax activists are, however, not only portrayed as victims, but also as members of a heroic resistance. Identity claims are thus spread by publishing the names of those who have decided not to be vaccinated, who are presented as critically minded citizens who pose themselves questions, who are healthy and pay taxes, the defenders of the constitution, peaceful demonstrators, those who disobey ('who do not want to bow their heads'), who struggle for freedom, who are dissidents. In a further step on from this, activists frame themselves as the unvaccinated that will save the planet, as being just as heroic as the antifascists during Mussolini's regime (i.e. the university professors that refused to swear loyalty to the regime are cited), who are prepared to lose their jobs in defence of free choice and free opinion. They talk of them-selves as true democrats, those who 'wait outside for the return of democracy', resisting unjust and illegitimate decisions and defending human rights and civilization, just like the courageous (suspended) medical doctors or heroic anti-Green Pass workers. In some versions of these identity frames, they are portrayed as 'true Italians' and/or true Christians (it is noticeable that the latter express support for Pope Emeritus Benedict XVI as opposed to Pope Francis I, who they at times consider to be an impostor).

A widespread definition of the self is aimed at a representation as loyal citizens who are unjustly discriminated against. A typical example of this nar-rative can be seen in the comment section under the *Commissione Dubbio e Precauzione, 'Nota del 2 gennaio 2022. Sul dovere di difendere lo stato costi-tuzionale'* (In Difendersi Ora 2022), where, after strict policies were adopted on the requirements of vaccination certificates to access public transport as well as various activities, a user wrote:

> these most recent decisions damage both our human dignity and our status as citizens. We pay taxes. And despite having paid subscriptions to museums and the-atres, we find ourselves excluded from everyday life. We no longer have rights and are no longer able to decide anything. Anyone who has a house on the islands will no longer be able to reach it even if they pay the taxes required for the property ... we are even isolated from friends and relatives, modern-day wandering Jews, we are living through an absurd situation from which nothing and no one seems pre-pared to save us ... We are the victims of a social experiment that would not have taken place if people had preserved and nurtured something very important over time and that is their self-awareness and awareness of their rights.

Unvaccinated people are thus framed as a repressed minority. In a post enti-tled *'Immunizzati alla democrazia'*, uploaded onto the website of the group Carmilla, an activist bemoans the fact that 'the area of opinion maliciously baptized "anti-vax", is the most vilified, mocked, denigrated form in the his-tory of the Republic, with millions of people who have felt insulted every day, for months, only because they are doubtful or reluctant to undertake a medical treatment that should be "free, aware and informed"'. In the same document, a persistent persecution is decried: 'as in all events in Italian his-tory, it begins with denigration by the editorialists and ends in anti-terrorism, a passage of which the first signs have been seen' (Iozzoli 2021).

Through the frame of discrimination, restrictions placed on unvacci-nated individuals are attacked as being oriented towards 'dividing society' by fuelling internal cleavages within the population. An activist, in his post

'*Sulla coercizione liberale*', elaborated on this by claiming that 'if you do not get it [the vaccination] you are singled out as a traitor, an enemy of the country, an idiot, a paranoid, ignorant person, an egoist, and a loser, thus fuelling the hatred and contempt of others' (Zhok 2021b). In fact, he adds,

> European governments today are competing with each other to invent new forms of harassment against the new public enemy number 1: the unvaccinated. … This morbid discriminatory logic, which violates a whole series of human rights that were believed to be 'inalienable', pits citizens against each other and will surely be described one day by historians as a kind of collective madness orchestrated by people who had lost all sense of democratic values and human rights.
>
> (Zhok 2021a)

Against this background, the resistance of the repressed minority is considered as heroic. Rejecting the widespread critique of anti-vaxxers as selfish individualists, activists represent themselves as the defenders of collective rights (Maccentelli 2022). With an assumption of personal responsibility for one's own health and defining themselves as 'resisters of vaccination and the Green Pass', anti-vaxxers praise themselves as defending their own body against a biopolitical authority. Care for one's own immune system is linked to individual choice. In this sense, the progressive, feminist movement slogan regarding the right to choose how one's own body is treated is appropriated for use against compulsory vaccination, which is defined as violating the freedom to make choices about one's own body. According to the same activist, the struggle therefore has a collective claim: 'not only does the defence of one's own body become the defence of many bodies and an expression of a collective idea of society where an authority considered illegitimate cannot claim the right to blackmail individuals or force them to have compulsory health treatments' (ibid.).

Against the assumed complicity of official experts, references are made to a few 'counter-experts'. The 'unique way of thinking of the regime virologists' is considered as based on the censorship of Nobel laureates such as Luc Montaigner, or well-known microbiologists such as Didier Raoult and dozens of other scientists they claim have been silenced by the mainstream.

As part of the assumption that 'the genetic serum does not immunize individuals', in an increasingly conspiratorial vision, the unvaccinated are defined as those resisting a capitalist plot. More specifically this resistance is aimed against 'a global plan that the power centres of capital at an international level have implemented operationally following the financial bubble at the end of 2019, in the context of a wider capitalist crisis and progressive monetary hypertrophy'. The activists point to the 'relationship between the crisis of capitalism and the biopolitical use of covid to manipulate the markets as a countertrend to the crisis itself, which by now has become quite serious and irreversible'. Resistance to the 'biopolitics of control and restrictions aimed at restructuring value chains' is thus considered to be part of:

> the class struggle between capital and labour, between the implosive model of rotting capitalism and vast masses of the people without mediations and social pacts in search of libertarian life paths through a generalized rebellion. A liberation of one's own bodies, of the freedom of movement, of refusal to be subjected to selections, discrimination, algorithmic tracking, evaluations, filing, inhibitions, prohibitions, which have exceeded the limit of a recognized and accepted normality.
>
> **(ibid.)**

In this vision, the 'popular resistance' is in fact defined as expressing a 'class struggle' in which 'the political avant-garde, just as has historically been the case, has the task of overcoming the barriers of an economism in workers "struggles and of politicizing them"' (ibid.).

Over time, isolation can be seen to feed a definition of the self as belonging to a persecuted and suffering group that heroically fights even when faced with extreme social stigmatization. In a speech at a demonstration on 15 January 2022, a 'coup disguised as a health intervention, a subversion of the foundations of the republic' was criticized by those who presented themselves as representing

> the teaching class that does not bow to the dictatorship, that which claims the right to work but also to decide on one's own body... And here we are, now. Take a teacher, with a single-income; after three months spent laboriously booking and taking covid tests for himself and his family, all of which had to be paid from his modest salary; now in December he learns that the sacrifices he made to keep the job that he loves, so that all the experience gained over the years would not go to waste, have been in vain because if he is not vaccinated he will still be suspended ... We go out into the open to melt fear like snow in the sun and remember that if a man is not willing to take any risks for his ideals, either his ideals are worth nothing or it is he who is worth nothing.
>
> **(Redazione Coordinamento Istruzione per la Libertà 2022)**

Conspiracy beliefs, therefore, fuelled sectarian attitudes. Thus, another activist evoked the 'Deep State', in a post in which he described the dark future he believed awaited the heroically resistant minority:

> we just have to force ourselves, tighten the bonds between us even further, pre-pare ourselves for the rapid deterioration of rights for those who continue to refuse brands, cards, conditioned 'social credit' cards, which will become our technocra-tized avatar. We will reject digital identity, which will be the only one that the State recognizes, and thus we will become bodies without rights, an irresponsible bur-den in the eyes of the inept democrats, the global uninformed, the collaborators who believe themselves to be 'responsible' and who will single us out for public mockery, as the source of all evil. And so, when our destiny is fulfilled, you will find me on the street, with a sign around my neck reading 'No QR Code', begging for survival.
>
> **(Franceschini 2021a)**

In summary, the identity framing combined the claims of a victimization of the unvaccinated with a vision of a heroic minority, endowed with a knowledge of absolute truth, resisting the attempts to impose a dictator-ship. Over time, there was a spread of increasingly pessimistic visions, with appeals to build secluded communities of the elected few in the name of the unvaccinated.

Oppositional frames: The global elite and their servants

Identity framing is closely connected with oppositional framing. In defining the movement identity as a resistance to a global plot, activists relate it to the framing of the enemy as the organizers of a conspiracy against the citizens. Indeed, it is noticeable that the oppositional framing points to the responsi-bility of a 'global elite' as well as their supposed servants. The former are part of a variegated list that includes 'Big Pharma', Bill Gates, global finance, the European Central Bank (ECB), the International Monetary Fund (IMF), the highest echelons of the state (accused of imposing digital identity cards), cor-rupt science, and so-called 'terrorist journalists'. These are all considered to be part of a plot by Western authoritarian capitalism and globalist technological capitalism. This alleged cabal is claimed to support 'authoritarian biopoli-tics' and whose eventual aim is to establish a 'communist sanitary regime' based on Chinese authoritarianism (part of what they term the 'chinesiza-tion' [sic] of society) and controlled by algorithms. Other political targets also include the Left, which is accused of betraying the oppressed, the 'anti-politicians' (including the Five Star Movement), 'a party on the opposition which is in government' (the League), as well as Draghi's 'government of the worst'. As part of this oppositional frame, corrupt politicians and virologists are denounced alongside journalists as 'globalists' and 'servants'. The framing also extends to the wider society, among whom the vaccinated are variously framed as zombies, anti-vax hunters, haters, drug addicts, and brainwashed individuals. In parallel, public opinion is depicted as being manipulated while religious targets include Pope Francis, who is defined as an anti-pope, leading a war against the Church.

In this highly conspiratorial vision, on a wider scale, global capitalist financial elites are claimed to have invented the pandemic in order to justify a Global Reset as, it is argued,

> Finance did not collapse because lockdowns had to be imposed; rather, lockdowns had to be imposed because finance was collapsing. The freezing of commercial transactions has in fact drained the circulation of money and the demand for credit. This has allowed for the restructuring of the financial architecture through extraordinarily aggressive monetary manoeuvres, which is only possible in the shadow of a stalled economy
>
> (Vighi 2021)

So, given an assumed acknowledgment of the 'impracticability of a liberal-democratic capitalism',

> The authoritarian management of the economy and society is imposed as a necessary condition for the (dystopian) survival of capitalism itself, which is no longer able to reproduce itself through mass wage labour and the annexed consumerist utopia .... The scenario that faces us, if we lift the veil of Maya, is of a markedly neo-feudal character. Less and less productive masses of consumers are regimented, simply because the new globalizers no longer know what to do with them. Together with the underemployed and excluded, the impoverished middle class has become a problem to be managed with the stick of lockdown (soon also in a climatic version), curfews, propaganda, and the militarization of society, rather than with the carrot of work, of consumption, of participatory democracy, of social rights (replaced in the collective imagination by the civil rights of minorities), and of 'well-deserved holidays' ... Operation Covid aims to safeguard economic privileges, not the health of citizens. Those who still persist in denying it become complicit in a system which, in order to survive, must terrorize.
>
> (ibid.)

The (vaguely defined) elites are accused of constructing the false narrative of a sanitary emergency in order to unleash unconstrained power. In Andrea Zhok's post, titled '*Infodemia istituzionale e stati ontologici dissociativi*', this group of plotters is singled out as follows: 'In the present pandemic circumstances something unprecedented has happened, namely the convergence of the highest political and media authorities in the production of a system of distorted, unreliable or undeniably false theses. ... in the midst of what should be a health emergency, therefore, guided by scientific precepts, we are swimming in a parallel reality based on the purest superstition'. The members of these evil forces are thus described:

> The first group is that of 'decision-makers', that is, those at the top level who bear full responsibility for having created this situation (the government *in primis*). The second group I would like to call the 'kapo' group, that is all of those who, although not part of the decision-makers, have taken enjoyment in exercising all of the power they were able to exercise to hurt, coerce, reject, denigrate and blackmail those who the 'regime truths' depicted as 'guilty'. For them, at least as far as I am concerned, there is no possible understanding, because whatever our 'information' is, one must always exercise a certain level of reserve on the human level before condescending to harm others, especially when they are in a position of weakness. ...
>
> The defence of the non-vaccinated against the assumed discrimination is so the basis for a denunciation of a 'moralistic power' accused of persecution of minorities, considered as impure, as in the totalitarian regimes of the past.
>
> (Zhok 2022b)

In an ever more sectarian opposition to this perceived total evil, it is politicians in particular, whether they have promoted or accepted policies aimed at reducing contagion, who are widely accused of having committed barbaric crimes. According to the *Comitato Liberi Pensatori*, for example,

> the introduction of the Green Pass by the Draghi government, which has now been extended to all workers, is a clear and vile case of blackmail, an attack on the freedoms and fundamental rights of man, a way of forcing the inoculation of experimental gene serums which have already either killed or made thousands of people sick, including many children! All of the parliamentarians who voted for him have been stained with a very serious crime and will have to be judged by the international courts as soon as possible in a modern day Nuremberg trial! We,

conscious Italians, have the duty to fulfil this mission and nothing will deter us from pursuing it.

(Bianco and Rotondo 2021)

A further oppositional frame accuses the Left of having betrayed its potential base. In this narrative, people queuing for vaccinations are described as representing 'a sociological cartography of modern power relations. We are all there, only because we no longer hold any kind of real power, not even that which can be exercised in the minimum essential space of our body, our blood, our immune system—what we would once have called an inviolable, natural, innate space'. In this situation, 'the problem is above all the lack of reaction on the part of that world of the popular left (or class, or alternative politics or whatever we want to appeal to, in our social or existential trenches), which is experiencing these epochal changes with very painful otherness', not seeing that

the 'pass' is not a provisional technical tool: it underlies a philosophy of governing things, a vision of the present, of the future, of the complexity that must be regulated. The Green Pass will become a lock pick—with unpredictable adaptations and methods—, a master key for all doors; a scheme to introduce 'a two-tiered citizenship', which is totally functional to the capitalist command.

(Iozzoli 2021)

Citizens in general are considered to be incapable of reacting to these plots. In a post in his blog, titled '*Sulla lettera di Cacciari e Agamben*', an activist denounced in the following terms the role of public opinion in what he defines as 'terrifying propaganda and moralistic pressure':

Precisely because it is fed by 100% of the media and 90% of the ruling political class, this 'moralistic suasion' has a frightening impact on public opinion. After having created a category of unvaccinated subjects (or perhaps vaccinated, but doubtful) as subhuman Anti-vaxxers, after having painted them as traitors to the homeland in the war effort against the virus, after having labelled doubters as carriers of death, it did not take long to reap the rewards in public opinion. These tones of apocalyptic moralism are the basis of a torrent of virulent hatred that can be seen on social media every day, where you find nurses who threaten to make unvaccinated patients pay, virologists who talk about the unvaccinated as mice that must be hunted out, doctors that wish them to suffer a death in their family, not to mention the infinite unending series of individuals who wish sickness and death on them.

(Zhok 2021d)

A similar tone can be found in a comment under the *Commissione Dubbio e Precauzione* blog on the responsibility of those who comply with the vaccination campaign, which reads: 'We must engrave the names and surnames of these traitors of the people, of the Republic and of the law in marble, so that the memory of this event remains alive until Judgment Day. May future generations remember these days as the days of infamy and spit on their graves' (Difendersi Ora 2022). Vaccinated citizens are thus presented as cowards:

A fictitious narrative has been prepared on the basis of a potential epidemic risk that is presented in such a way as to favour extreme submissive behaviour ... The multitudes exposed to media bombardment not only bend, but even self-discipline, adhering with grotesque enthusiasm to forms of civic duty in which coercion becomes altruism, to the point that the struggle for the common good has even resurrected the infamous practice of informing ... the cards on the table have been changed to legitimize the greatest vaccination campaign of all time, the absurdity of which can be summarized with the following question: why should the whole of humanity (including children!) inject themselves with an experimental serum with increasingly disturbing adverse effects that are outside the norm ... For the uninitiated, in Europe the digital health passport was scheduled to be introduced in 2018, with implementation scheduled for 2022.

(Vighi 2021)

It is not surprising that the oppositional framing on the Right of the political spectrum bridges heroism and victimization by the traditional array of enemies. In this case it is migrants and the politicians who defend them that are identified as being responsible for the lack of freedom. This can be observed in the call for a demonstration made by the radical right-wing organization Casa Pound, which stated: 'the enemy is those who promote liberticidal laws that have little to do with health concerns, blaming citizens who have already been crushed by an unacceptable increase in the cost of living for their failures'. In this narrative the punishment reserved for true Italians (i.e. unvaccinated Italians who presumably cannot take money from their banks

or are seen as 'prisoners' as they cannot travel without a vaccination certificate) is contrasted with what they consider tolerance for the 'crimes' of
migrants:

> While the police are busy checking Green Passes, the neighbourhoods, even those
> in the city centres, have become a land of conquest for bands of undocumented
> criminals who are free to roam about in all weather. While the government imposes
> limitations and restrictions on Italians, including restricting movement, our bor-
> ders are continually crossed by thousands of illegal immigrants. Our cities, and
> Italy itself, are hostage to a government of incompetent people who, in bad faith,
> feed a health emergency only so they do not have to address the real problems
> including that of illegal immigration.
>
> **(Lorenzo 2022)**

Over time, the definition of the enemy can be seen to take on an increasingly
antagonistic tone. On the websites of *Studenti contro il Green Pass* ('Students
Against the Green Pass), contributions denounce the various transformations
in the 'dictatorship that are needed to start a Great Reset', with government
policies even defined as the work of Satan. So, for instance, one activist
discussed his conversion to an anti-vax position as a religious conversion:

> With the advent of these experimental drugs I was not just convinced, but I was
> absolutely sure that the enemy was about to proceed in violating the precautionary
> principle and the Nuremberg Code … A confidence grew in me, and I understood.
> My research activities increased dramatically, and I dedicated all my time to it. I
> thought of the confinement, the curfew, the images of helicopters chasing citizens,
> the elderly separated from their loved ones … understood that a decision had been
> made to kill off a large number of people. I realized that I was dealing with the chil-
> dren of Satan. I observed the horror and had the courage to continue observing it.
> I immediately rediscovered God, as always. To choose God, for me, is to hope in
> Jesus Christ. I must hope to be on Christ's side, to ensure the immortality of my
> soul. I must hope for the immortality of my soul in order not to suffer the greatest
> evil of all, which is the horror of emptiness.
>
> **(Studenti contro il Green Pass 2022a)**

In short, the oppositional framing pointed to a cosmopolitan elite that
exploited the pandemic for their material profits and power, but also, more
generally, to those who collaborate with the elite (such as national politicians, journalists, medical doctors, and scientists), or just comply with orders.

With the passing of time, the frames singled out the vaccinated as the main opponents, who were not only accused of indifference to the suffering of the unvaccinated, but also of being a burden on the latter as a result of their assumed unhealthy habits.

Expanding the comparison: Anti-vax framing in Germany and Greece

Also in Germany, the diagnostic framing espoused the idea that compulsory vaccination was a goal sought by scientists and the rich, that science is manipulated, and that the virologist Christian Drosten and Bill Gates were their main enemies (Koos 2021). More so than in Italy, QAnon conspiracy theories (linked to paedophilia and satanism) were found to be widespread, with the frequent use of slogans such as 'Save the Children' and 'WWG1WGA' (Where we go one, we go all). Puzzlingly, while the New Age wing presented itself as linked to nature, the presence of climate change deniers and supporters of the 'Great Replacement' conspiracy (including right-wing exoteric activists at war with Satan and the anti-Christ) was not contested from inside (Wetzel 2021; Benz 2021a; Benz 2021b). In addition, ultra conservative religious milieus promoted circles of 'concerned parents' against vaccination as well as against gender rights, spreading fake news relating to the presence of foetuses in the vaccines. The anti-vaxxer's criticism of the media has been summarized as follows: 'First of all, the "mainstream media" are one-sided because, in their view, "critical" experts are not present. Second, the media would portray the Corona protests in a defamatory and distorting way. Third, like politicians, they would stir up fear' (Frei and Nachtwey 2021: 19).

In an often instrumental way, the presence of the Far Right notwithstanding, from the outset of the pandemic there has also been a very prominent and persistent equating of the anti-contagion measures with the actions of the Nazi regime, which

can be seen in the talk of the 'conformist press' or the 'Enabling Act' with reference to the Infection Protection Act, but also in the secondary anti-Semitic self-staging of the protesters as victims with 'non-vaccinated' Jewish stars or in the identification with protagonists of the resistance against 'National Socialism' … Symbols of Nazi resistance and liberal democracy, e.g. Sophie Scholl or the Basic Law, are appropriated and filled with new meaning

(Teune 2021)

Moreover, adapting to specific episodes in German history, the organizers of the anti-vax protests also framed them as resonating with the 1989 movement for democracy against the authoritarian regime of the GDR. The demonstration in Leipzig in November 2020, for example, was staged as a historical re-enactment of the Monday Demonstration on 6 November 1989 that preceded the fall of the authoritarian regime, repurposed as 'Angela Merkel: "it is Your 1989"', which was announced on posters and in memes.

As for the prognostic framing, various streams of protesters converged on a highly individualistic conception of freedom, which was particularly evident among the New Age milieu. Extreme forms of individualism were combined with an attempt to present the fight against vaccination as similar to the fight against authoritarianism in the GDR (Benz 2021a). Activists promoted a

> libertarian understanding of freedom which set self-determination and personal responsibility as absolute value … In their individualism, there is a pronounced tension with a state perceived as strongly antagonistic, which interferes with their own way of life, even when this serves to protect others. In their exaggeration of their individualism, they are directed against socialization, but not against communitarization in specific milieus and self-organized contexts
>
> **(Frei and Nachtwey 2021: 24).**

In addition, anti-vax, far-right frames are bridged with the claim of national sovereignty against presumed conspiracy against the fatherland. On 29 August 2020, for example, the Far Right protested at the statue of Frederick the Great on Unter den Linden in Berlin, with posters bearing slogans such as 'Not built for slavery', 'The only thing evil needs to thrive is for good men and women to remain silent. Rise up!', and 'GDR 1989 = FRG 2020'. On the same day, activists displayed posters in black, white, and red which read 'We summon the Emperor.' Between a US flag and a Russian flag, a poster read: 'Trump versus Warmongers Capital Crimes on Children! STOP Fake News Media Lying Press—911 INSIDE JOB War on Terror'. Protestors also stated, 'we, the people, are sovereign and a peace treaty must be made'. A slogan was: 'Germany Supports Donald Trump and the Citizen of the Republic for the USA. Stop the Morgenthau Plan!' (Hanloser 2021: 192).

A common feature in the identity framing of anti-vax protestors in Germany was the narrative of the protests as going beyond the Left and the Right. If the concept of *querdenker* would seem to hint at an attitude somewhere between new thinking and questioning, it is clear that anti-vax activists were more likely to believe in conspiracy theories spread through the use of digital technology (Reichardt 2021; Pantenburg, Reichardt, and Sepp 2021). While research on German anti-vaxxers singled out a widespread mistrust of science, activists, however, presented themselves as open-minded individuals, who listen to both sides of an argument but trust their feelings (*Bauchgefuel*), believing they have good intuition, all the while lamenting the divisions in families and friendship circles caused by debates on Covid-19. Anti-vax activists, who were generally from older demographic cohorts, highly educated, and middle class, declared themselves to be the victims and expressed a keen interest in fundamental rights.

Paradoxically, while anti-vaxxers compared their discrimination to that suffered by the Jews during the Nazi period, there was also a significant proliferation of anti-Semitic conspiracies even beyond the far-right environment (Volker 2021). While citing Sophia Scholl as a hero of the resistance against Nazism, anti-vaxxers promoted demonstrations against 'Zionists, Satanists, transhumanists and pharmamafia' (Balandat, Schreiter, and Seidel-Arpaci 2021: 106). In fact, various streams saw a convergence around radical right-wing framing, which often also incorporated conspiracy beliefs as well as open support for Trump as a saviour for humanity. While 'trust, love and freedom' were initially the main slogans in one of the first protests in April 2020, one of its the main promoters, Michael Ballweg, used symbols from the QAnon conspiracy theory as early as August. At these protests there were also groups of supporters of Donald Trump.

Called by the self-defined *Querdenker*, the events were presented as rooted in the 'heroic capital' of the 1989 movement for democracy; a 'Friedliche (R)Evolution' (peaceful (r)evolution) was proclaimed, with the aim 'to repeat history together'. The far-right frames also brought about exclusive forms of nationalism, with patriotism counterposed to globalism. Its leader defined the protest in Berlin on 1 August 2020 as being characterized by 'patriotic critique of globalism and its control of the media world' (Sellner 2020; Virchow and Häusler 2020).

Turning now to Greece, it can be observed that the ultra-nationalist milieu used Covid-19 conspiracy narratives to frame the pandemic as part of a plot to defy the rights of the indigenous natives to self-representation.[5] A group calling themselves 'Indigenous Greek Natives' expressed their opposition to 'Whichever intervention against the Individual Freedom of Greeks by officials of the state, laws or anything that is NOT related to their personal assets, e.g. the use of masks, self-testing, rapid-tests, molecular tests, compulsory

---

[5] The reconstruction of the Greek case is based on the research report by Stella Christou (2022).

vaccination, removal of organs, compulsory issuing or exhibition of medical documents, special permits, fines, taxes (with no exception), restrictions,
closure of businesses etc.' Promoting a similar position, the 'Custodians of
the Constitution' appealed to the idea of patriotic self-defence, stating that
the vaccination campaign would destroy the native Greek genetic code and
threatening harsh punishment for those who promoted vaccination:

> In the face of the violent and illegal infringement on human rights with the purpose
> of the genocide of the nation of the Greeks and the extinction of the physiology
> and uniqueness of its genetic code through the violent vaccination of the whole
> population, in spite of national resistance. AFTER THINKING ACCORDING TO THE
> NATURAL LAW AND IN THE INTEREST OF THE NATION OF GREEKS. I forbid the intro-
> duction and the use of mRNA vaccines. ... Those that, despite this prohibition, dare
> to use the vaccine as well as those that have introduced it, will lose their political
> rights, their nationality and their citizenship, they will be banned from the country
> for life, or they will be punished with life imprisonment without the right to change
> the sentence irrevocably.
>
> **(cited in Christou 2022)**

In the diagnostic framing, antivax groupings in the New Age milieu combined conspiracy theories about the vaccination with the chemtrail conspiracy. This theory has been spreading since 2003, with a peak in 2013 when,
according to data published in the newspaper Ethnos, 33% of the around 1000
respondents agreed with the statement that 'they are spraying us [with chem-
icals]'. As in the Italian case, small groupings attacked anti-contagion policies
as being oriented towards controlling citizens and forcing blind obedience.
This is made clear in a document calling for a demonstration in Athens, in
which the 'Initiative against the health Apartheid' called for a defence of the
'body' from 'experimentation':

> The imprisonment (*egkleismos*), the movement restrictions, the prohibition of
> political gatherings, the lay-offs, the compulsory vaccination and the unprece-
> dented violation of rights, are not characterized by [concerns for] healthcare but
> aimed to meet the needs of the new normality imposed by the restructuring of
> capital, the overcoming of the capitalist crisis and the violent paradigm shift. No
> to compulsory vaccination, direct or indirect. Vaccination is a personal affair, not
> a means to divide and exclude. We should not allow our body to become the field
> of experimentations of pharmaceutical [companies] and biotechnology [industry].
> No to the display of healthcare certificates, no to the utilization of humiliating

'privileges'. The [collective] mobilization by orders of the state is not 'social solidarity' or 'class duty', it is complicity. Solidarity with those that have been fired
and those that have been suspended due to their refusal to subject themselves to
compulsory medical procedures! Resistance to the blackmail, the indirect reduction of wages through compulsory tests and the monitoring of our health by the
state and bosses!

(ibid.)

Vaccination is thus considered to be part of a plot designed by the bio-
pharmaceutical industry to weaken natural immune systems and thus create
greater dependence on drugs. According to a post created by the group
behind the 'Sarajevo Magazine' on 31 March 2022:

The destruction of the natural (human) immunity and of the natural immune system IS NOT some sort of 'mistake' or some sort of 'accident' in the epic march
of techno-science and 'progress'! On the contrary: it is a fundamental method to
create permanent dependence of the population on the designs and the products of the health industry as part of the 4th industrial/ capitalist revolution. After
having established a polarity in agricultural production [based on the idea that]
'each year we sell the genetically mutated variety of plants together with its next
disease so that we have permanent clientele', the biotechnology of the big chem-
ical/pharmaceutical companies, through the imposition of genetic engineering as
the 'only therapeutic possibility' (in the contemporary capitalist world), (where it
could) has made the last jump of profiteering and control of the human species. ...
[By] hacking the immunity system, a permanent morbidity (personal and collective) is produced—the permanent morbidity (which is attributed to anything
else but genetic engineering!) requiring permanent or repetitive (genetic) 'thera-
pies'. The health industrialists hate health but, together with their shareholders,
adore the perpetual profits and perpetual control of 'labour'—as is 'natural' for
capitalism, is it not?

(ibid.)

As part of this narrative, then, people are said to be obediently subscribing
to 'suicide' as well as to the 'invisible mutilation' of their immune system.
The consequence of this willingness leads to profits for their killers, which
is something that they cannot see as they have been blinded by the propaganda of 'death sensationalism' and the campaign of terror orchestrated
by government officials and the mainstream press. Conspiracy theories have
also been supported by a number of members of the Greek parliament, such
as Rachil Macri (who moved from the Independent Greeks party to Syriza

and subsequently to the anti-vax, right-wing party, the Free People). With an extremely abstruse narrative, which mixed an assessment of the 'killing' effects of vaccination with religious mysticism, the physics professor Giorgos Pavlos argued that:

If we let children get vaccinated then they enter into a process [whereby] in the recent years they will get sick with cancers, strokes etc. This game is so smartly designed that people do not realize it. As a scientist I have sat down and examined all of the existing studies and I am convinced, and this is why I am speaking out publicly and say that this vaccine is a murderer. It is a biological weapon, an experiment that is being carried out on humanity and we do not know where it will lead us. Those that get vaccinated have fallen into a trap because they have believed in a lie. The fact that they force you to put substances that you do not know into your body, is in itself a crime. No one should accept this. No one can impose on an individual the right to do anything to their body. We have to protect our body like we protect our churches. We should not allow any doctor or politician to touch our body in this brutal way. In this moment, Greece, where journalism has collapsed, vaccines have arrived to finish off the Greek people. It is worse than what happened in 1940, than what happened with the genocides. Now this is happening to the whole of humanity. Any scientists that support this project are complicit in a crime. They should be tried and must be put in prison.

(ibid.)

As s mentioned, as with Catholic fundamentalism in Italy, one element that is particularly specific to the Greek case is the involvement of parts of the Orthodox Church in the anti-vax campaign. These elements have promoted conspiracy theories that see the Covid-19 pandemic and anti-contagion measures as the work of Satan, oriented at establishing a New World Order. This theory has been especially spread among the 'Friends of Elder Paisios' (a monk, living at Mount Athos, who died in 1994 and became a saint in 2015), whose Facebook pages have promoted anti-vaccination positions. Building a catastrophic vision, a video (with 150,000 views) claims that decades before the pandemic, Paisios had written that:

Things are progressing as usual. In the US dogs that are locked up emit signals through their transmitters and, tac, they find them. As such, they know where each dog is. Any dogs without chips, any stray dogs are killed using laser beams. And then they'll start killing people. Tons of fish have been branded ... Now again a new disease has appeared, for which they have found a vaccine which will be compulsory and through which they will brand them [the receivers]. How many people are already branded with laser beams, some on the forehead, some on the arm! Later, whoever has not been branded with the number 666 will not be able to sell or to buy, or take a loan, or to be appointed [to a position the public sector] etc. My mind tells me that the Antichrist wants to trap the whole world in this system, and if someone is not in the system they will not be able to work etc, whether they're red, or black or white, it is everyone. In this way a new economic system with be established, that will control the global economy, and only those that have received the brand, the etching with the number 666, will be able to make market transactions. But what will happen to those who get branded! I was told by an expert that laser beams cause damage. Those people who will be branded will attract the rays of the sun and will be so damaged that will chew their tongues from the pain. Those that are not branded will be better off than the rest, because Christ will help those who are not branded!

(ibid.)

While more embedded in broader New Wave and Far Right groupings in Germany than in Greece, in both countries conspiratorial framings spread with a radicalization over time towards a dichotomic vision of absolute good and absolute evil.

Conclusion

As has been outlined in this chapter thus far, the frame analysis dealing with the Italian case has demonstrated that there was a bridging of different collective frames during the anti-vax protests. With regard to the diagnosis of the problem, the two sets of frames addressing, respectively, the danger of the vaccines for individual health and the danger that the management of the pandemic posed for democratic developments and citizens' rights, merged into a narrative in which the pandemic is mainly seen as instrumental in the establishment of a global biopolitical power. In terms of prognostic framing, the solution to controlling the virus (which is defined as mild) is located in alternative cures and a generic return to a *status quo ante*, which is promoted as the minimal common denominator. Calls for freedom are bridged with those for national sovereignty. Identity framing is subsequently oriented towards linking a presentation of anti-vaxxers as victims of a 'sanitary dictatorship' that turns them into 'second-class citizens' with that of heroic freedom fighters resisting powerful elites. As part of the oppositional framing, the latter are thematized as an oligarchy, promoting a global conspiracy with the support of corrupt politicians, fake experts, and a mass of zombie servants. In different contexts, anti-vax protestors called for constitutional freedom in the face of an assumed dictatorship.

The comparison of the Italian case with the German and the Greek contexts confirms some shared characteristics of the anti-vax framing. Notwithstanding some differences, there is a convergence of Far Right and New Age milieus on regressive frames that promote individual freedoms as absolute values, with little concern for solidarity with those more exposed to the virus, who are considered as responsible for their own destiny. On this view, the Far Right had already bridged its frames with those of religious conservative milieus during anti-gender campaigns with a commercialized New Age milieu, which had moved towards a focus on self-optimization. The spreading of conspiracy theories helped the convergence of diagnostic, prognostic, identity, and oppositional frames around the sectarian counterposition of absolute good and absolute evil, with spirals of growing isolation.

In conclusion, the framing of the antivax movement is characterized by the connection of a range of prominent narratives, originating in various milieus, which share a view of the world that is heavily based on conspiracy beliefs. The racist and ultra-nationalist visions of the Far Right and the individualist beliefs of the New Age milieu are bridged with a narrative of biopolitical authority. In this fashion, the pandemic is considered to be a plot designed by global elites, aimed at implementing a 'Great Reset', by inventing a virus and, especially, by using vaccination as a means to acquire control over the bodies—or, more specifically the DNA—of the subjects, who are thus deprived of all of their rights. As in many sects, anti-vaxxers present themselves as a small minority, heroically resisting an almighty enemy. Conspiracy elements imported from various sources are combined with each other, triggering increasingly self-referential dynamics.

Although it facilitates convergence between different groupings and provides the true believers with shortcuts to assess emerging and unknown threats, as is the case within sects, conspiracy thinking does not, however, seem able to sustain mobilization or support long lasting commitment. As has often been stressed in research on framing dynamics, in order to mobilize, frames should be credible, both in their content and in their sources. Incoherent messages, or messages originating from actors that are either unknown or have a questionable reputation are unlikely to elicit the same reception as messages from actors with a respected public image. Frames should also be salient, by touching upon meaningful and important aspects of people's lives and show high 'narrative fidelity' (Benford and Snow 2000). Most importantly, however, they should resonate not only with their targets, but also with the broader cultural structure in which a movement develops (Williams 2004:

105–8). The alignment between the frames of movement activists and those of the wider population is a condition for mobilization, which is achieved through the integration of their mobilizing messages with widespread beliefs among the population to which they are addressed. An important condition for the spreading of protest is the frame bridging between the representations articulated by movement organizers and the interpretations of reality held by large sectors of public opinion.

Vice-versa, when there is a large distance between activists' frames and those present in the rest of society the result is a reduction in the potential for symbolic re-elaboration (Swidler 1986). This is the case in the framing of the anti-vax protests, which is characterized by increasing references to obscure conspiracy theories. While conspiracy beliefs may be widespread among the population, their resonance would seem to be hampered by the fact that they are commonly stigmatized in the public sphere. A further aspect that reduces the credibility of the frames is the incoherence of the conspiracy theories on which they are based, as well as the questionable reputation of the actors promoting them. This is contrasted with widespread evidence for the lethality of the virus and the effectiveness of vaccination, as well as the narrative fidelity in terms of confirmation in everyday experience, which has contributed to greatly reducing the spread of anti-vax discourses. All of this is compounded by the vicious cycles that are typical of sectarian dynamics, in which isolation pushes activists towards increasingly conspiratorial narratives that in turn produce further isolation (della Porta 1995). A final, but not insignificant, factor is the fact that the increasingly threatening narratives employed by anti-vax activists contribute to the spread of fear, which has proven to be a problematic emotion for mobilization. Additionally, in a depoliticized environment, any attempts at the politicization of vaccination hesitancy proves an arduous task.

Indeed, it seems that the conspiracy narratives investigated here were unable to resonate with a large part of the population. In particular, neither the previous waves of protests against the vaccination of children and seniors nor the 'sovereigntist' forms of exclusive nationalism spread beyond small circles. The same is true for the radically anti-state narratives, which can be seen to have been imported, together with QAnon conspiracy theories, by both the Far Right and the New Age milieu. It is particularly noticeable that all of these narratives seemed quite at odds with the growing demand among the population for state intervention to tackle the spread of the virus. They did succeed, however, in increasing anxiety in a context of uncertainty.

5

Anti-vax Protests and Social Movement Studies

Some Conclusions

In this volume, I have used a number of major concepts in social movement studies to investigate the protests that emerged during the pandemic in opposition to policy measures that governments at different levels introduced in order to reduce contagion. While at times also mobilizing in order to claim economic compensation for forced inactivity or investment in social services and education in order to allow for a selective and secure reopening, most of these protests ended up targeting Covid-19 vaccines.

More generally, the pandemic has seen very different types of protests. On the one hand, progressive social movements have mobilized in defence of social rights and participatory democracy. In different forms—including innovative repertoires of protest in the street but also initiatives practicing mutual help and the development of alternative knowledge—progressive social movements have called for and produced solidarity by bridging claims on social and environmental justice within a broad call for health rights (della Porta 2022). On the other hand, disruptive protests have mobilized loose coalitions of far-right, anti-EU, ultraconservative Christian, New Age, and anti-vax groups that have targeted the measures taken to mitigate infection, up to and including the very denial of the existence of a pandemic. Regressive framing focused on the defence of individual freedoms, with an actual denial of solidarity with the part of the population that was most exposed to the virus and its consequences. As part of a neoliberal vision, health was considered as a personal responsibility to be achieved through alternative practices and compliance with the so-called natural order. Over time, protests were fuelled by and contributed to the spread of conspiracy beliefs that had already characterized regressive politics.

In general, in the Global North the organizational resources for the anti-vax protests came from a tried and tested alliance of far-right movement organizations and parties, including ultraconservative religious fundamentalist

Regressive Movements in Times of Emergency. Donatella della Porta, Oxford University Press. © Donatella della Porta (2023).
DOI: 10.1093/oso/9780198884309.003.0005

positions, with a New Age component that, although originally close to environmentalist networks, had recently moved towards apolitical stances within an individualistic conception of freedom and commercialization especially around alternative health treatments as well as education. While there were regional differences in the balance between these components, over time a leading role, at least from an organizational point of view, was assumed by the far-right groupings, who employed a narrative that was increasingly influenced by conspiracy beliefs, in particular the QAnon and Great Replacement plots. While part of the organizational resources mobilized in the anti-vax protests come from previous mobilizations against vaccination, the narrative developed towards a sectarian discourse that pitched absolute good against absolute evil, spreading fear of a dictatorship that aimed to carry out an anthropological transformation within a 'Deep State', a message resonant with that developed by the anti-gender movement (Prearo 2020; Lavizzari 2021). In the New Age milieu, small groups had previously mobilized, especially against policies relating to the compulsory vaccination of children through campaigns that have at times been supported by public funds (particularly in the United States under the Trump administration) as well as generous private funders. With a convergence of exoteric and religious conservatism, structured around anti-science and anti-state positions, fake news, and conspiracy thinking spread on social media, but also through in-person events, in particular around the broadcasting of a documentary film with unsupported claims about the effects of vaccination (Rohlinger and Meyer 2021). Indeed, past experiences have shown that conspiracy theories and New Age ideas often developed in synergy with each other (Asprem and Dyrendal 2015). The term 'conspirituality' has been used to point at the convergence of conspiracy beliefs and New Age holistic thought in a hybrid system that combines emphasis on the self with conspiratorial visions. Conspirituality has been presented as 'a rapidly growing web movement expressing an ideology fueled by political disillusionment and the popularity of alternative worldviews', which 'offers a broad politico-spiritual philosophy based on two core convictions, the first traditional to conspiracy theory, the second rooted in the New Age: 1) a secret group covertly controls, or is trying to control, the political and social order, and 2) humanity is undergoing a "paradigm shift" in consciousness' (Ward and Voas 2011).

Targeting lockdowns; curfews; social distancing; the compulsory use of face masks; the requirement to be vaccinated, recovered from Covid-19 infection, or to have tested negative for infection in order to enter public spaces and access certain locations, up to and including compulsory vaccination; these protests came to be known as anti-vax. Although they did not always explicitly mention vaccination, the protestors shared a vision of the virus as a rather mild disease and the consideration of anti-pandemic measures (including vaccines) as not only being of little use, but also posing a danger to the bodies and the minds of citizens, even viewing these procedures as the expression of a full-fledged 'dictatorship' put in place by shadowy forces. While far from representing all non-vaccinated people, or even all of those who were critical of government pandemic policies, the protestors claimed to act in the name of those who refused vaccination. Even if they only involved a tiny part of the population, the anti-vax protests were able to attract a great deal of attention, if only for a relatively short period of time.

While often presented as heterogeneous in their social and political composition, anomalous in their ideological profile, and pre-modern in their repertoires of action, I have suggested here that these protests can be considered to be a form of regressive contentious politics during an emergency critical juncture. Indeed, in line with the conceptualization of right-wing thinking, they privileged individual freedom over equality, as well as personal interest over the common good. They were also anti-modernist in nature, aligning on anti-state positions. The mobilization was logistically supported by a Far Right that had undergone a transformation during the Great Regression, with the spread of nativist positions linked to anti-EU 'sovereigntist' frames and ultraconservative religious values, in conjunction with a New Age milieu in which hedonistic and individualistic positions had grown with increasing commercialization. There was also a significant retrograde character to the protests, with anti-vax activists constructing a dystopian view that was heavily influenced by politicized conspiracy beliefs in the plots of Satanist cosmopolitan elites drinking the blood of innocent children. The QAnon conspiracy was bridged with other conspiracies relating to chemtrails and 5G that had previously been widespread in the New Age milieu, those surrounding the 'Great Replacement' of the white, Christian race widely shared on the Far Right or those on the use of aborted foetuses for the production of vaccines that were common among fundamentalist Catholics. Over time, conspiracy frames fuelled a sectarian closure around increasingly abstruse beliefs in cruel dictatorial plots and self-victimization. Spreading through a connective logic of action based on a crowdsourcing model, the anti-vax protests did create some convergence between different actors around a regressive vision; however, their capacity to embed themselves in resilient networks, while varying by location, tended to remain low.

The empirical research presented in this volume has provided an in-depth analysis of anti-vax protests in Italy, which has been analysed as a critical case not only due to the fact that it was the country in Europe, and the Global

North more widely, in which the virus spread first and with most dramatic consequences, but also as it was the country where anti-contagion measures have been most severe. In addition, the research has compared the anti-vax protests in Italy with those in Germany and Greece, considering the former as a case with high levels of protest diffusion and the latter as a case of limited diffusion. This cross-national comparison, which has been expanded through secondary literature, highlights not only the similarities present in the different contexts, but also the impact that national mobilizing structures and protest opportunities had on the intensity and the forms of the anti-vax protests.

In this concluding chapter, I first aim to summarize some of the main empirical results on the repertoires of action, organizational models, and collective frames in the anti-vax protests, initially in Italy and then from a comparative perspective with the other case studies. Furthermore, I will connect these characteristics of regressive movements to general and country-specific opportunities and challenges for anti-vax protests as well as their expected societal impacts. In doing this, I will locate the empirical results within general reflections on the effects of emergency critical junctures, such as the Covid-19 pandemic, on contentious politics with particular attention to the transformative role of protests, i.e. their capacity to trigger new forms of action, organizational models, and collective framing. In the final section, I will reflect on the sectarian evolution of anti-vax protests fuelled by vicious cycles as well as their potential consequences.

The mobilization resources of the anti-vax protests

Research in social movement studies has stressed the importance of resource mobilization as intervening between structure and action, but also between individual frustration and the collective responses to said frustration (della Porta and Diani 2020). The analysis of anti-vax protests in Italy has indicated a number of trends that seem to be shared across many countries. In particular, it can be seen that the anti-vax protests built upon previous experiences of mobilization during the so-called backlash (della Porta et al. 2022), with conspiracy beliefs being adapted to counter awareness of environmental challenges (such as global warming) as well as attacking civil rights (within racist and anti-gender campaigns). Far-right activists, interested in expanding their constituency, engaged with a New Age milieu in the area of alternative health practices in which hedonistic values had spread together with a commercialization of activities and a belief in conspiracies (among others, on the use of chemtrails or 5G as instruments of total control). To differing extents in different countries, it was regressive movements that were leading the anti-vax protests. While they varied in strength, these anti-vax mobilizations remained, however, episodic, fragmented, and were not sustained over time. This research has therefore attempted to explain both the rapid spread but also the swift decline of the mobilization.

Looking at the Italian case in depth, the protest event analysis has helped to disentangle the general characteristics of street politics and the dynamics of different waves of contestation that form broader protest cycles. Generally speaking, the number of participants at marches and static demonstrations tended to be small, with events mainly organized at a local level. Larger marches at a national level were rare events, and usually targeted new policy measures aimed at controlling the evolution of the pandemic during peaks in infection. Overall, the anti-vax protestors mostly failed to mobilize a social base of those most affected economically by the pandemic. The number of events fluctuated, becoming more intense during rising waves in the spreading of contagion, and were more frequent in the capital and in the largest cities in the north of the country.

Within these general trends, two waves of protests were singled out in the Italian case. While in 2020 and in the first months of 2021 there were protests especially by social actors that felt more impacted by the anti-pandemic measures and called for state support, the anti-vax and anti-Green Pass protests only grew (and then quickly declined) during a later phase, from the summer of 2021 onwards. In fact, the main actors involved in the two waves remained mostly separate, even though in both instances the Far Right, including religious fundamentalist and ultra-nationalist, anti-EU groupings, provided organizational resources as well as collective frames for the mobilization.

During the first wave of the pandemic, beginning in the spring of 2020, workers in a range of sectors asked for more, rather than fewer, anti-contagion restrictions, including better preventions in the workplace. A number of protests against a second lockdown were subsequently called in the autumn of 2020 by obscure social media channels that especially addressed employers and employees in the service sector (particularly in tourism) who had greatly been impacted by the pandemic. Given the limitations on organizing marches, the main forms of action were sit-ins, which were often combined with symbolic performances. Students, their parents, and their teachers also used forms of direct action (such as connecting to online classes from the streets in front of their schools) to call for a reopening of in-person didactic activities. Artists developed creative forms of protests, especially in the form of cultural performances in order to ask for public

support for cultural activities. In these cases, the claims were for the investment of public resources that would compensate for economic losses related
to the pandemic as well as for the reopening of some specific spaces and
activities in a secure fashion. These requests were subsequently negotiated,
with some success, by traditional interest groups (such as unions and business associations) as well as newly founded grassroots organizations (such as
Priorità alla Scuola, a group formed by teachers, parents, and pupils).

Although they declined during the first half of 2021, protests re-emerged
in the summer of 2021, this time targeting the vaccination campaigns in particular. Unable to involve those individuals who had been economically most
heavily hit by the pandemic, protests against anti-contagion measures instead
mobilized the anti-vax milieus, where contacts had already developed in previous waves of contention between the Far Right, including ultraconservative
religious groups and anti-EU nativist parties in particular, and a commercialized and hedonistic component of the New Age milieu built around
alternative health and educational practices. The protests were mainly called
by local coordination committees, with an unstable convergence of previously existing anti-vax groups within a New Age milieu, anti-Europe parties,
and anti-gender groupings mainly located on the Right, with a notable
presence also of the more traditional Far Right. While the widespread stigmatization of these protests apparently discouraged broad participation, the
spreading of conspiracy theories—such as the QAnon conspiracy—allowed
for a convergence of the anti-state and anti-modernist views present in both
milieus. Some attempts at national coordination, through groups such as
Coordinamento 15 Ottobre, *Basta Dittatura*, and *Fronte del Dissenso*, had limited success as they were characterized by reciprocal competition and internal
divisions.

Especially from the autumn of 2021 onwards, a radicalization process was
visible in certain cities around (often unauthorized) marches. Initially, as
protestors defied the rules that were in place both to reduce infection (i.e. by
refusing to wear face masks and maintain physical distance) and to manage
the organization of public demonstrations (about which the local authorities
must be informed of in advance), the police at times intervened to identify, fine, and even arrest participants. Given the existence of restrictions on
protests or on carrying out protest in certain places, the violation of the orders
of the public authorities brought about an escalation, as the police intervened to clear public spaces and disperse the marches. A number of more
violent events took place in Rome, especially in the autumn of 2021 (including the attack on the headquarters of the main trade union, the CGIL, and
the attempt to place government buildings under siege) and subsequently in

Trieste (with the occupation of a number of docks and street battles with the police). Following these episodes of violence, stricter rules were introduced against the Saturday afternoon protest events periodically called in several Italian cities, leading to stricter police controls and a steady reduction in the number of protestors.

From a symbolic point of view, the protests remained linked to traditional forms of sit-ins initially and subsequently marches, with the development of a specific choreography that was very resonant with that which had previously characterized the anti-gender protests. As revealed by the video analysis, while Italian flags were commonly used, posters and speeches made frequent reference to a Fascist dictatorship (to which the Italian 'regime' had been assimilated) as well as to the Holocaust and the victims of the Shoah (with whom the protestors liked to compare themselves). The demonstrations, which were mainly made up of small groups of middle-aged individuals, tended to fade away in the space of a few months, while calls for hunger strikes, legal challenges, and roadblocks failed to mobilize a volatile base.

The organizational structure of the anti-vax protests tended to follow what I have defined as a *disembedded crowdsourced model*, characterized by a reliance on online appeals for the self-mobilization of a constituency that was, however, weakly networked and remained highly fragmented. The emerging movement organizations mainly remained localized, with a number of short-lived coordination committees at a city level, and a proliferation of small groupings (at times with overlapping members and little more than a social media account), operating through the creation of online platforms that distributed toolkits for different activities. Social media remained the main channel used to promote protests through the online distribution of forms of instructions for self-mobilization as well as how to document the protests. Thus, various grouping not only published toolkits online for organizing demonstrations, but very often also templates for legal challenges that individual activists were called on to use against specific anti-contagion policies (from face masks to vaccination certificates) with particular advice for specific professions (from those in the health sector to those in education). There were lawyers present in several of these groupings, as well as the (very small) number of anti-vax personnel in the health sector, who also provided advice about diets and natural products to be used in order to cure or even prevent Covid-19 infection. A similar crowdsourced model was also used by several tiny parties and electoral lists that distributed instructions on how to meet and form local chapters on their online platforms.

The wave of protest also remobilized groups that had survived from previous mobilizations against compulsory vaccinations by adopting more formal structures (including groups advocating for home schooling and those in the commercialized New Age milieu), but also from anti-EU campaigns, claiming to fight 'globalism' and to defend national sovereignty, as well as related neoconservative and far-right organizations. In strong tension with the calls against a supposed dictatorship, the presence of the Far Right is especially evident in the appeals to national sovereignty, within a quite exclusive definition of the Fatherland (visible, among other things, in constant presence of Italian flags). On the Far Right, splinter groups and tiny parties bridged the narrative of a global conspiracy with exclusive forms of nationalism and contrasted the supposed heavy hand used by the government against the anti-vax protesters and unvaccinated autochthonous Italians with the alleged tolerance shown towards migrants, which they singled out as the real danger. Often aligned on anti-vaccination positions (at times based upon fake news claiming the presence of foetuses in Covid vaccines), anti-gender groupings provided a mobilized base, often aggregated in Church spaces, and a choreography based on the stylization of protesters as victims of a cruel dictatorship aimed at destroying religion. While the anti-vax protestors stressed a call for the defence of constitutional freedoms, the alliance with the Far Right, including anti-gender groupings, favoured a convergence towards anti-democratic conceptions of freedom as a sort of individual natural rights.

Crowdsourcing, however, was unable to sustain mobilization in the long term, given the weakness of individual and collective ties. While there was often a reliance on online platforms for the preparation of demonstrations or the establishment of political groupings, attempts at coordination never stabilized. Various media platforms, from local outlets to national television channels on YouTube, blogs to Facebook posts, and, in particular, Telegram accounts, shared texts and images that spread conspiracy theories and fake news relating to the virus and the anti-contagion measures. However, this developed into a very closed environment for members of the in-group, with the creation of an abstruse language that was more oriented towards the consolidation of the sect than towards communication with the outside world. Moreover, the unselective use of social media provided the police and the judiciary with information on illegal activities (which included the above-mentioned break-in at the headquarters of the main Italian trade union, the crowdsourced map of commercial activities not requiring customers to show a Green Pass or the harassment of experts, journalists, and politicians).

While some symbols and idols were often imported from abroad (especially from the United States and Germany), the organizational structures remained extremely fragmented, with internal division between those more focused on the building of some forms of isolated communities of self-proclaimed experts and those who instead wished to engage in political activity. Fights also developed among these two components, especially as the mobilization declined, with party lists particularly in open competition with each other, while personal conflicts and small group dynamics further increased fragmentation. In this sense, a very liquid structure, composed of loose nets, mainly connected online, showed low levels of resilience when the reactive dynamics against anti-contagion measures were blunted, following the decline in the severity of the pandemic thanks to the actual roll-out of vaccination. Attempts at repositioning the anti-vax groups into a pro-Putin front during the war in Ukraine had a very low mobilizing capacity. It is particularly noticeable that while the presence of the Far Right was not considered as problematic by the mobilized activists, it most likely discouraged other networks from joining the protests (e.g. certain squatted centres or environmental groups), who had expressed criticism of vaccination and the vaccination pass but refused to ally themselves with reactionary actors.

Notwithstanding the diversity evident among the mobilized groups, in action, the collective framing became quite homogeneous, especially among the hardcore protestors during the last wave of mobilization in autumn 2021. While in the first wave claims were more pragmatically oriented to put pressure on decision makers to provide economic support and to undertake public interventions in order to allow for the reopening of certain activities, during the second wave, frames were bridged around conspiracy beliefs that clearly dominated the definition of both the problems as well as of the solutions, with the adoption of narratives that had been developed abroad, especially in the Alt Right in the United States, tied to various versions of the QAnon conspiracy that, having also emerged in the United States, had penetrated different milieus well beyond the Far Right.

The diagnostic frames focused on the denigration of the vaccines, which were considered as not only of little use, but also as dangerous. The 'genetic serum' was accused of producing long-term negative side effects in the bodies of vaccinated individuals, triggering a wide range of diseases from blood clots to various types of cancers. Additionally, the vaccines and vaccination certificates were considered as means for imposing total control over the vaccinated population. The agents of these plots were defined as a global elite, which was led by Big Pharma and included at its apex political and economic leaders (often of Jewish origin) as well as international institutions such as the World Health Organization and the World Economic Forum, among others. Helped by their 'servants', such as journalists and experts, this elite was considered to be intent on not only increasing its profits and power but also, in the most extreme versions, reducing overpopulation by killing many innocent civilians through the use of vaccines and face masks, thus saving capitalism through a so-called 'Great Reset'. Racist conspiracies, such as the claimed 'Great Replacement' of the white and Christian population with migrants of colour and Muslim background were also mobilized, as were those relating to the use of chemtrails and the 5G network as instruments of domination.

The prognostic framing showed retrograde and dystopian characteristics. While the vision of the future remained underdeveloped—aside from general appeals to a return to the world as it was before the pandemic or to 'nature' and a more 'human' life—the prognostic framing also follows conspiracy beliefs in its vision of a heroic (and, at times, victorious) resistance of the oppressed, which was mainly identified as the non-vaccinated population. As victims of a 'sanitary dictatorship' that had transformed them into 'second-class citizens', the non-vaccinated are presented as the ones who will save the world from the 'vaccinated zombies'. The return to national sovereignty in the face of globalism is linked with a proclaimed defence of the supreme (Western) value of individual freedom. Indeed, anti-vaxxers considered themselves to be freedom fighters who (like the partisans that fought against the Fascist regime in Italy) were courageously resisting a powerful and evil elite, or would at least survive by building autonomous communities. While making an appeal to alternative 'experts' and attempting to argue for some of their claims through the extensive use of data (from dubious sources), the conspiratorial narrative and the aggressive language strengthened both fear and insecurity. The main shared components in the framing process have been a strongly individualistic conception of freedom, as well as anti-modern and anti-state positions. As mentioned above, the idea of victimization as well as the denunciation of a presumed 'dictatorship' broadly resonated with the language that had been previously developed by anti-gender groupings (Lavizzari 2021).

As previously mentioned, anti-gender protests, which had developed in opposition to activism on women's and LGBTQ rights and its deconstruction of an essentialist vision of gender and sexuality, combined with a call for natural law, which resonated in anti-vax conspiracy thinking. In both, the claim of resisting attempts to curtail the freedom of speech of members of a 'silent majority', who are self-represented as victims of discrimination, is accompanied by attacks on equal access to rights by LGBTQ individuals and women, and even goes as far as a rejection of laws against violence towards women and sexual minorities (Bracke, Dupont, and Paternotte 2017; Mayer and Sauer 2017). The self-presentation by anti-gender activists as the protectors of innocent children against the egotism of adults intent on organizing a marketing of said children and as defenders of human rights are further elements that resonate with the anti-vax narrative (Ayoub and Stoeckl 2023). Similarly, something that is resonant with the anti-vax discourse is the fear of a secret plot by the alleged supporters of gender ideology, defined as an anthropological and epistemological threat to Christian values.

While claiming to defend a culture of life against the culture of death, the anti-gender protests, in a similar fashion to the anti-vax events, expressed the fear of losing ethnic, religious, and racial privileges. Emerging from the discursive radicalization of the Catholic associations that focused on the 'defence of the family', anti-gender groups opposed, just as anti-vax movements have, the assumed 'anti-naturalist' secularist positions, considering the Cairo Conference on Population and Development in 1994 and the fourth Conference on Women in Beijing in 1995, which established the right of women to control their reproduction capacity, as opening an anthropological challenge to 'naturalist' position based on essentialist visions of sexual identities (Lavizzari and Prearo 2019). As has been seen in the anti-vax protests, also in the anti-gender ones there is a mirroring of feminist discourse through resignification—in what is defined as a battle of the nation against the fraction, and of the public interest against the lobbying of organized minorities (ibid.: 101). Irrational instincts and individualistic interests are considered to be terrifying characteristics of a 'gender fluid generation', while, as with the anti-vaxxers, parental education is considered as an inalienable right in the face of state interference. A further element that anti-gender groups share with anti-vaxxers is, in fact, the spreading of a moral panic (more specifically a 'gender panic' or sexual panic) against what they claim to be a challenge to human anthropology, as biological sex is seen to form the basis of the natural family. There is not only opposition to specific gender rights but also a denial of the epistemic approach to these rights (Lavizzari 2021).

In a similar fashion to the anti-vax events, the anti-gender protests have been also characterized by systematic ties with the Far Right, with overlapping narratives on anti-globalism, anti-EU positions, nostalgia for a lost golden age, and the scapegoating of various types of minorities (Paternotte and Kuhar 2018). In fact, just as in the anti-vax mobilizations, in the anti-gender action campaigns converged under the protection of international allies, globally spreading and nationally adapting repertoires of contention and framing through various forms of cross-national diffusion (Ayoub and Stoeckl 2023). Influenced by the '*Manif pour tous*', which emerged in 2012 in France and was imported into Italy, where it then peaked with the Family Day of 2015, the *Popolo delle Famiglie* (People of the Family) and related groupings have consolidated their links with the Far Right (Lavizzari 2021). Not only did several of these groups support anti-vax positions and participate in anti-vax protests, but the repertoire of actions of those protests were resonant with the mix of flash mobs, conferences, lobbying, and widespread use of social media that was noted in relation to the anti-gender groups in the past (ibid.).

The anti-vax protests from a comparative perspective

To summarize, with regard to the Italian case, research on the repertoires of action, organizational structures, and collective framing of the anti-vax movement has indicated an escalation in the forms of contention, which became increasingly frequent from the autumn of 2021 onwards. This can be seen in the street interactions with the police, increasing sectarian trends within the crowdsourced organizational models, and the convergence on a call for unrestrained freedom mixed with conspiracy theories as master frames for the mobilization.

Many of these characteristics were also confirmed by the analysis of the German and the Greek cases, albeit in different combinations and with a number of specific elements. The similarities between the case studies may be linked to the shared challenges as well as the transnational spread of slogans, symbols, and narratives, which was facilitated by the global nature of the pandemic crisis that, naturally, constituted the common context for the anti-vax protests in the various countries examined. However, the observation of country-level specificities makes it possible to better understand the general dynamics of the anti-vax protests in relation to available resources and opportunities.

As far as the *repertoires of action* are concerned, the protest cycle in Germany tended to last longer than in Italy or, even more so, than in Greece. Beginning at a very early stage in the pandemic in the south-western region of Germany, the protests soon extended to most states in the country. The mobilization started as early as the beginning of the first lockdown within the New Age milieu, which saw a swift commercialization of the *Querdenkers* protest brand. The protests spread through the use of a large (albeit loose) social media net, starting with quite large national demonstrations in Berlin as early as August 2020, when the presence, if not the prominence, of the Far Right became gradually more visible, only to soon become dominant. This was particularly the case as the protests spread to the eastern states. Although the visibility of the Far Right had the effect of reducing sympathy in public opinion, it did not, however, discourage alliances with an exoteric milieu into which QAnon symbols and narratives had already penetrated.

Radicalization came about very early in the cycle, especially with the previously mentioned attempt to storm the Parliament in Berlin on 29 August 2020, which in terms of the slogans and symbols employed, was quite reminiscent of the Far Right–led protests in the United States that had climaxed in the armed storming of public buildings. This radicalization continued into later stages of the pandemic during interactions between protestors and the police, as protestors defied anti-contagion rules (especially relating to face masks and social distancing) and subsequently resisted police orders to disperse. Even when resorting to so-called 'promenades', aggressive behaviour towards journalists and the police was often noted. An even more aggressive example of intimidation was seen in the pickets placed in front of the private houses of politicians and the harassment of doctors and journalists— all of which were actions that had been called for online in an anonymous fashion. The protests remained sustained during the winter of 2021, in parallel with the waves of the virus, with several national events taking place as well as coordinated protests in several German cities involving hundreds of protesters.

Conversely, in Greece, protest was very rare and mainly consisted of small demonstrations. While some contestation of anti-contagion measures was organized by the Orthodox clergy (based on a rejection of state intervention in Church matters) or libertarian groupings (opposing restrictions on individual freedoms), protests were rare events due to efforts at an institutional level, supported by both the government parties and the opposition alike, which were aimed at reducing the spread of the virus as well as any related disruptions to the tourist activities that form an important element of the economy of the country. Opposition to anti-contagion measures, which was supported by individual politicians and entrepreneurs already well known for their conspiracy views, remained weak, with a number of sporadic national events taking place in the second half of 2021 when vaccination became compulsory for certain professions and age cohorts.

The anti-vax protests were also characterized by confrontational strategies in other countries. In general, it has been noted that the contentious repertoire included actions of disruption or obstruction of sites for vaccination and other public health facilities, harassment of doctors and politicians, but also refusal to wear masks and keep social distance or to show proofs of vaccination when required (Snow and Bernatzky 2023). In the United States, 'Many of the protests feature demonstrators wielding semi-automatic rifles and other firearms, meant as symbols of popular sovereignty against the perceived oppression of government elites' (Stavrakakis and Katsambekis 2020: 55).

As far as the *organizational structure* is concerned, in anti-vax networks, based on disembedded crowdsourced models of collective action, were joined by far-right activists. In Germany, as in Greece, the protests mobilized resources from an unstable convergence of far-right activists with nativist nationalist groups as well as a New Age milieu with individuals and enterprises involved in alternative medical and educational practices, including anti-vax groups that had formed in opposition to previous vaccination campaigns. Religious fundamentalist groups were present in both. One of the main differences in the organizational composition of the protests was the significant presence in Germany of a relatively large New Age milieu, which had lost its connection with the environmental movement and had become ever more commercialized, as seen in the spread of anthroposophical institutions and related business products. Moreover, following a short period in which it had called for harsher anti-contagion measures, the main far-right party in Germany, the AfD, became very supportive of the anti-vax protests, providing a significant amount of organizational resources and political support especially, but not only, in eastern states.

In contrast to this, in Greece the New Age milieu remained marginal, with the environmental movement maintaining progressive positions and rejecting conspiracy beliefs relating to 5G technology or 'chemtrails'. With the main far-right party, the Golden Dawn, in disarray, and a right-wing national government, the mobilization only found support on the Right in very tiny ultranationalist groupings. In a context in which ambivalent positions were initially taken by the religious leadership of the Orthodox Church, anti-vax activists also mobilized some components of the lower clergy. However, the protest organizers appeared to be loosely coupled and weak in terms of mobilization capacity. What is more, the reliance on social media for crowdsourced campaigns, which was a similar factor in both countries with appeals to self-organize, could not sustain the protests over time, instead leading to the development of sectarian dynamics.

In other countries the organizational structure of anti-vax campaigns also fits the *disembedded crowdsourced model* that I have singled out in the Italian case and confirmed in both Germany and Greece. In the United States, for example, the anti-vax movement has also been described as made up of 'an extensive organizational bedrock consisting of a network of loosely coupled national and statewide nonprofits, private organizations, grassroots groups, and celebrated figureheads' (Snow and Bernatzky 2023: 189). While the Covid-19 pandemic has increased trust in science among the largest cohort of the public opinion, it has also consolidated anti-vaccine beliefs among those activists who were already committed, offering various occasions for mobilization against the increasing spread of pro-vaccination policies. During the waves of protest at different stages of the pandemic, the anti-vax core has been hybridized with other components, involving far right-sponsored conspiracy networks in particular. Indeed, the anti-lockdown protests, sparked by the shelter-in-place orders oriented towards slowing down the transmission of the virus, were described as populated 'by a variety of actors, including anti-maskers, long-gun toting militia types, flag-flying supporters of the Confederacy, anti-vaccination adherents, and folks pressed to get back to work' (Snow 2023: 513). While not necessarily adhering to the Far Right, it is also the case that in other countries the other anti-vax groups did not attempt to distance themselves from them, calling instead for the 'old' Left–Right divisions to be overcome.

As for the *collective framing*, a very similar approach was adopted in Germany and Greece, with the assumed ineffectiveness of the vaccines, or even the danger posed by them, forming the basic narrative that was promoted in order to attack the vaccination campaigns that it was claimed were part of an evil plot. Face masks and social distancing were equally considered to be instruments for the imposition of total control by a dictatorial power, in which national politicians were involved alongside prominent (often Jewish) individuals, such as Bill Gates or George Soros. The World Health Organization as well as national virologists were accused of spreading fear around what was claimed to be merely a flu-like virus. In both countries, moreover, globally spread conspiracies were bridged with national ones, such as those involving the domination over the German or Greek people. Specific historical experiences—such as the authoritarian regime in the German Democratic Republic or the austerity crisis in Greece—were also referred to by ultra-nationalist groups on the Far Right in order to claim revenge for historical injustices. In Germany, in particular, the QAnon conspiracy was spread by far-right activists with the aim of claiming a role as 'concerned parents' intent on protecting children against alleged attacks by migrants. Launched in 2017, the QAnon conspiracy travelled to Europe towards the end of 2018, initially through the UK, and subsequently to a massive extent in Germany—so much so that in 2020 and 2021, messages in German relating to the conspiracy were more widespread than those in English (Scott 2020; Hoseini et al. 2021). The far-right Reichsbürger movement, which was particularly active in the anti-vax protests, attempted to bridge the QAnon narrative with the claim that the Federal Republic of Germany is an illegal and non-sovereign state that had neither signed a peace treaty after the Second World War nor adopted a constitution, calling on Donald Trump to sign a peace treaty.

In Greece, conspiracy beliefs were especially widespread in the small network of anti-vax activists. Alongside individual promoters of fake news, a number of Orthodox clerics also opposed mask-wearing and vaccination, and even participated in protests together with the Far Right, spreading conspiracy fantasies relating to satanic plots ('They're implanting chips with 666 by vaccinating us') and disobeying state regulations which limited the use of the churches in order to reduce infection (FES Friedrich-Ebert-Stiftung 2021).

More generally, in both countries, as well as in Italy, the organizers of anti-vax protests often appropriated different frames in order to bridge various existing or desired constituencies—from neofascist to anti-gender groups, and from anti-EU to the New Age factions. Research carried out on various countries has in fact pointed towards a sort of usurpation of symbols from other movements, including progressive ones. In a study on communication in online forums such as Facebook groups, parenting sites and Reddit subgroups, it has been noted that anti-vaccine narrative is based on a rhetoric which is

> directly appropriated from other sources, ideas or movements that provoke strong feelings. … one constant is the use of language that has been repurposed from other divisive debates. Families invoke 'natural parenting' in worrying about the long-term effects on their children of a new vaccination technology. Political activists speak of 'medical freedoms' and of personal rights to choose what goes into their bodies. Freethinkers who distrust authority figures in government or academia are inclined to 'do their own research' or discuss conspiracy theories. The religious bring up the idea that some vaccine ingredients may violate Jewish, Muslim or Hindu dietary restrictions.
>
> (Goyal, Hegele, and Tenen 2021)

Within the appeal to freedom and the denunciation of evil elites, traditional anti-vaccination claims have also been updated in other countries and spread worldwide: this can be seen in calls for 'freedom of choice on medicine' in opposition to a supposed 'medical dictatorship'. More generally, Snow and Bernatzky (2023: 188) have distinguished six mobilizing diagnostic frames against vaccination, with claims that '1) vaccines are unsafe; 2) vaccines are ineffective; 3) mandatory vaccination is a violation of personal freedom and parental and medical rights; 4) vaccines are fundamentally compromised by pharmaceutical interests and governmental corruption; 5) the science surrounding vaccines is either theoretically misguided, tainted or not yet good enough; and 6) vaccines are rendered unnecessary in the face of natural immunity and a commitment to holistic living'. As they have noted,

> The relative salience of these frames has varied temporally with variation in the social and political context and the movement's trajectory. Initially, the dominant frame emphasized the health dangers and risks of vaccines, but when legislative initiatives began to mandate vaccination and constrain personal and medical exemptions, the rights and personal freedom violation frame moved center stage with its emphasis on parental and physician rights. This shift in no way suggests that anti-vaccine adherents are less concerned about the safety of vaccines, but instead are deliberately and strategically shifting their framing away from an overt discussion of the effects of vaccines to the right to refuse them. Overall, these six frames reflect deeply rooted anxieties about risk and safety, longstanding political tensions between individual and collective freedoms, and the holistic lifestyles that continue to draw people into the vaccine issue.
>
> **(ibid.)**

Indeed, during the Covid-19 pandemic, a commonly shared master frame has been embedded in a narrative that contrasted the dangers of vaccines with the efficacy of alternative health practices. In the United States in particular, the rejection of vaccination was motivated by the denial of the seriousness of the virus, which was bridged with various conspiracy beliefs relating to a plot by shadowy elites against the people as 'the anti-lockdown protestors shared in common a burning disdain for institutionalized expertise and governmental authority, mocked communal rights in favor of individual rights and liberty, and were mainly Trump enthusiasts' (Snow 2023: 513).

In general, the main aspiration in the framing of the anti-vax protests was backward looking, namely the reestablishment of a lost order. Anti-lockdown claims aimed at abolishing lockdown, anti-mask claims aimed at withdrawing the obligation to wear masks, and anti-vaccination claims targeted the use of vaccines and the vaccination certificate. The rationale provided was that there was no health emergency, but rather a plot concocted by a cosmopolitan elite against ordinary people oriented towards the establishment of a 'New World Order' or a 'Deep State'. In this discourse, 'the libertarian defence of personal freedom over government is often tied to reactionary demands for law and order, threats of violence, and displays of sheer cruelty asserting that the economy was more important than health' (Gerbaudo 2020: 69). In Denmark a (weak) anti-vax movement also developed around the image of freedom fighters challenging state totalitarianism (with Danish politicians accused of being almost like Nazis). Displaying Danish flags, the protestors stated that, 'There is a war between the elite and the people, and if you are angry and upset it is because you are being attacked every single day' (Garcia Agustin and Nissen 2022: 751). In this direction, anti-vaxxers called for 'a return of the "old normal", a reversal to the pre-pandemic conditions, starting from the most obvious everyday life elements, such as the ability to move freely without wearing a mask and abiding by other anti-contagion regulations' (ibid.).

Anti-statist, far-right frames bridged with anti-gender and anti-vax narratives, in particular, travelled from the United States to Europe, following the entrepreneurial investment of economic resources. Generally speaking, the anti-vax movement remobilized international connections from previous campaigns against vaccination. To cite just one example, among those invited to the demonstration in Berlin on 29 August 2020 (as well as to several other protests in Europe, including in Italy) was Robert Francis Kennedy, Jr., a nephew of John F. Kennedy, who had spread fake news claiming that there was a link between vaccination and autism (Virchow and Häusler 2020). The same individual also participated in anti-vax rally in Italy.

The organizers of the anti-vax protests often claimed to be part of the chosen few who possess knowledge relating to the 'truth', presenting themselves as 'sober experts and courageous resistance fighters at the same time'. Thus, a proto-scientific style based on self-taught expertise has been singled out, as anti-vaxxers considered themselves to hold on to their expertise even in the face of social ostracism, stigmatization and repression: 'As initiates they have the truth, as resistance fighters they hold on to it publicly' (Frei and Nachtwey 2021: 18; see also Eisenmann, Koch, and Meyer 2021). Comparing organizations spreading conspiracies over Covid-19 vaccines, Drążkiewicz (2022) had shown how these groups appropriated and imitated methods associated with civil society, with mimesis and mimicry employed as strategies that contributed to their survival and expansion. While at the same time courting, coveting, despising, and dismissing the authority of medics and scholars (Song 2010), groupings bridged anti-vax conspiracies with anti-gender and anti-migrants ones, albeit imitating scientific jargon and claiming the support of experts, to varying effects. In Poland, where a divided society has previously seen Catholic priests and right-wing politicians lend their support to the spread of conspiracies at various points in its history, a number of Catholic bishops and several conservative organizations expressed doubts about compulsory vaccination, and some went as far as to spread the false narrative that Covid-19 vaccines contained the cells of aborted foetuses (Drazkiewitz 2022). In Ireland, a consensual society in which anti-vaxxers enjoyed no political support, their attempts to mimic scientific rhetoric and present themselves as representing society as a whole largely failed (ibid.).

In practice, the reliance to a greater or lesser degree on conspiracy theories produced an anti-vax narrative that was based upon a sentiment of fear. While the slogans used appeared to contrast negative sentiments (see, for example in the organization of 'No fear days'), while media and politicians were accused of spreading terror, it is the very conspiratorial narrative itself that projected the terrifying scenario of a 'Great Reset', the end of democracy, and the death of society. As has been noted, 'the movement propagates "Don't be afraid" (of the virus); often stickers with this slogan were distributed on the fringes of the demonstrations. At the same time, however, the "Corona rebels" are pursuing a very determined fear policy' (Hanloser 2021: 206). Suffice it to recall that one of the most widespread and terrifying fantasies was the idea that the virus was created by the WHO in order to reduce overpopulation.

Fear was also spread by the QAnon conspiracy theory, which has a number of specific characteristics in terms of both its content and format. In late 2017, the anonymous user 'Clearance Patriot Q' started posting messages on 4Chan, a platform often used by conspiracy theorists and far-right radicals. The main thrust of the story they propagated was that Donald Trump was fighting a war against a 'Deep State' lead by cosmopolitan elites (ranging from the leaders of the Democratic party, including Hillary Clinton, to Hollywood celebrities and billionaires), who were devoted to Satanism, Vampirism, child-trafficking, and paedophilia. Pretending to be a government insider, 'Q' posted cryptic 'Q-drops', claiming that certain, seemingly incomprehensible statements made by the US president Donald Trump, the paladin of the fight against the supposed cabal, could be understood in light of his revelations (Murru 2022). According to QAnon, 'influential, global satanic elites would kidnap, torture and murder children in order to extract a rejuvenating drug from their blood. With the image of the bloodsucking elite, this completely insane narrative draws deep from the arsenal of vampiristic-anti-Semitic, incidentally also sexually neurotic lust-fear fantasies' (Hanloser 2021: 207). Indeed, the Jewish Rothschild family was presented as leading the satanic cult as well as depriving non-Jewish citizens of their property. If fearful individuals are more prone to believe in conspiracies (see below), a highly politicized and threatening conspiracy theory like QAnon, actively promoted by the Far Right, penetrated the New Age and Christian-fundamentalist milieus (Virchow and Häusler 2020). Groups of followers subsequently used Facebook and YouTube to elaborate on the Q-drops, introducing new talking points (Scott 2020).

In terms of format, QAnon is based on an *open* combination of narratives and characters typical of the conspiracy imaginary (such as Satanism, paedophilia, ethnic minorities, etc.) with emerging elements (such as gender and the pandemic), which are located within 'an over-arching frame that places each of them within a clear plot of destruction and redemption' (Murru 2022, 165). As a *politicized* conspiracy, it locates contemporary political developments within the Manichean vision of an ongoing battle between Good and Evil. From an *improvisional millennialism* perspective (Barkun 2013), the expectation is put forward that the struggle will end with the victory of the righteous and the defeat of the corrupt elite. A sudden political storm will lead to the triumph of the Good, with the arrest of the paedophile Satanists and the return to the founding values of America: 'When the time is right, Q will give the signal, and the people will rise and join Trump in the showdown against the forces of darkness' (Murru 2022: 165). The conspiracy theory is explicitly *right-wing* as it considers a far-right populist such as Donald Trump to be a heroic fighter against the cabal of progressive cosmopolitan Vampirists, thus combining 'most disparate religious, secular, scientific and political elements united under the power of a controversial leader' (ibid.).

What is more, the QAnon conspiracy is based on an *open narrative* which is constructed through crowdsourcing, as 'QAnon storytelling relies less on compact and exhaustive ideological frames and more on anonymous, ephemeral, cryptic drops that are written in a way that spurs readers to fill in the blanks left in the narrative' (ibid.: 166). Through this *crowdsourced* process, political developments are integrated into the narrative alongside emerging facts (such as Trump's electoral defeat) without challenging the vision of the apocalyptic battle led by a super-hero. QAnon entrepreneurs, from far-right activists to professional communication experts, use *multi-media channels* to disseminate the conspiracy theory to different audiences, adapting the style of the communication to the characteristics of the various platforms. QAnon messages thus spread in a complex network including Youtube videos, Reddit boards, Facebook groups, Telegram chats, and chan forums, which are often strategically infiltrated by the far-right activists. Additionally, the selling of various gadgets or tickets to QAnon events makes for a high economic profitability (von Nordheim, Rieger, and Kleinen-von Königslöw 2021).

Thus, the dissemination capacity of the QAnon-linked conspiracy narrative can be seen to be related to its network form, which increases its viral speediness through conspiratorial hermeneutics (Hannah 2021). The defence of traditional family values, which is particularly appealing to religious fundamentalism, is promoted within the conspiratorial narrative by QAnon's vision of women as centred on motherhood and maternal duties: 'Whether it is by collaborating with strangers in a QAnon affiliated social media group to decipher the latest "Q-drop" or calling the National Human Trafficking Hotline to report that online retail giant Wayfair is actually a front for the cabal's global child sex trafficking ring, women engaged in the QAnon movement are able to assert their feminine identities as protectors of the innocent and regain a sense of maternal efficacy' (Bracewell 2021). In general, through *cross-national diffusion,*

> QAnon has also developed locally, hybridizing with the conspiracy themes and anti-government rhetoric already established in pre-existing conspiracy subcultures. QAnon has therefore become a 'blurred conspiracy theory', diluted and fragmented into isolated pieces. Without its original cohesiveness, the QAnon theory has become a generic symbolic referent for bigger and obscure plots in which some people are secretly pulling the strings in what the mainstream thinks is reality. In this second form, concepts and narrative frames originating from QAnon have been mixed up with pre-existing conspiracy theories (such as those related to vaccines, 5G, Soros, Bill Gates, etc.) and fully adapted to the local conspiracy milieu.
>
> **(Murru 2022: 173)**

In summary, the symbolic and actual radicalization in the forms of action; the weak mobilization capacity of the crowdsourced model given its lack of deep-rootedness in society; the conspiracy narratives; and the language that was increasingly oriented towards insiders all combined to introduce sect-like developments within the anti-vax movement through spirals of isolation. The regressive characteristics of the anti-vax protests also became more and more evident in the affiliation of the mobilizing networks with the Far Right, as well as in the focus on an absolute defence of individual freedoms and the disregard for solidarity with those groups who were potentially most at risk of contracting the virus and/or suffering the worst effects of infection. In general, individualistic views were reflected in a conception of health as a personal rather than a collective responsibility.

Anti-vax protests in emergency critical junctures

When exploring the historical conditions for the development of the anti-vax protests during the Covid-19 pandemic, the characteristic of said health crisis must be considered in depth. As explained at length in the introductory chapter, I have considered the protests against anti-contagion measures as regressive forms of contentious politics in an emergency critical juncture (see also della Porta 2022). Characterized by rapid and quick changes that deeply affect everyday life, fuelling discontent, which may in turn be mobilized in collective action, contingent on their development and open-ended in their effects, critical junctures are particularly influenced by the types of actors that mobilize on specific claims. The first truly global pandemic had, however, very different and very localized characteristics (Bringel and Pleyers 2020; de Sousa Santos 2020), which also affected contentious politics.

As an emergency critical juncture, the pandemic disrupted peoples' lives, triggering various types of grievances. The anti-vax protests targeted, in particular, what activists defined as restrictions on individual freedoms. As mentioned in the introduction, there is no doubt that government policies oriented towards reducing infection were very intrusive. The Covid-19 pandemic was addressed through emergency measures that dramatically constrained the rights of movement, assembly, and expatriation. Research based on an analysis of over 13,000 Covid-19 policies worldwide has concluded that 'early Covid-19 policy responses across countries have been based on different kinds of policy mix dominated by authoritative policy tools— such as curfews and lockdowns, border restrictions, quarantine and tracing, and regulation of businesses' (Goyal and Howlett 2021: 259). In the EU, as many as fourteen countries declared a state of emergency at various points from February 2020 onwards, and five of them resorted to emergency powers (European Parliament 2020). As many as twenty-three European countries imposed restrictions on Freedom of Assembly and Association, and Freedom of Movement which had a widespread impact on other fundamental rights and democratic principles, such as the right to education for schoolchildren and the right to work for the many adults who lost their jobs (IDEA 2021a and 2021b). Freedom of expression and the holding of free elections were at times also challenged (ibid.). Even in democratic contexts, the health crisis deeply challenged public institutions on issues of legitimacy and efficacy (Offe 2021). States of emergency are however certainly contemplated by democracies, even if limited in time (White 2019). Anti-contagion limitations on individual freedoms were generally supported by public opinion as necessary in the pandemic conjuncture in order to save lives. Progressive social movements especially tended to call for strict measures in the name of solidarity with the weakest sections of the population, who were also those considered to be more at risk.

The increasing inequalities that came about during the pandemic are also relevant for a greater understanding of the anti-vax protests. Richard Horton (2020) has, in fact, used the term 'syndemic' to point to the synergies between the virulence of Covid-19 and the presence of other non-infectious chronic diseases, linked to weak primary prevention, pollution, and increasing inequalities in neoliberal capitalism. As Claus Offe (2021) has rightly noted, the position of each individual in relation to the virus varied vis-à-vis both the health hazard and the effects of lockdown measures. Thus, although 'for a moment, there was a sense of interdependency and unity ... after a few weeks of lockdown, the unity started to fracture' (Vandenberghe and Véran 2021: 181). The pandemic made the inequalities in the endowment of social rights more visible: from the very right to health coverage and sick leave (or leave to care for others who were sick) to the right to housing and access to public education or social services. The shelter-in-place orders increased the impact of unequal living conditions in relation to housing rights, discriminating against those who had either insufficient or no private space and little or no access to ever more important equipment such as computers or internet connections. The pandemic especially disrupted the most commodified educational systems, with dramatic consequences for students, teachers, and other workers in various roles. This fragmentation of individual positions during the pandemic was reflected in competing demands, such as those in secure employment calling for lockdown measures while those in insecure employment feared the potential consequences of such restrictions. While anti-vax protestors rarely succeeded in mobilizing the constituencies of those most severely hit by the anti-contagion policies, they did manage to spread appeals to the younger cohorts, pointing to the reduced health risks posed for them, as well as to the small businesses in the service sectors.

While these are general trends, when comparing Italy with Greece and Germany, considering different specific social and political developments can help to explain the different intensity and characteristics of the protests against anti-contagion measures. First and foremost, the higher intensity of protests in Germany (followed by Italy and Greece) can be connected with higher levels of 'liquid modernity', triggering among other things the spread of neoliberal individualist values in the form of personal 'self-optimization' (Rocke 2021). Related to this are visions of health as an individual responsibility linked to claims for individual freedom in the choice of health practices. Diffidence towards public intervention, which is widespread in the large New Age milieu, dovetailed with anti-statist developments in the Far Right. In both milieus, specific anti-vax conspiracies could be bridged with existing beliefs in a number of already present conspiracy theories about plots by a small (and evil) elite aimed at controlling the native population. A higher degree of digital hyperconnectivity in the former might have facilitated the spread of fake news and conspiracy theories, something that was also helped by higher levels of commercialization in the New Age milieu that supported anti-vax positions. While traditionally considered to be less trustful than Germans, Greek and Italian citizens showed instead less diffidence towards medicine and science.

What seemed to have been even more important is the different degrees of politicization of positions on anti-contagion measures. While in Greece, with the Golden Dawn in disarray and the Centre Right in government, support for anti-vax and similar positions was very limited, in Italy the League (which was in government for only part of the pandemic period) and the Brothers of Italy (who were in opposition) occasionally supported anti-mask and anti-lockdown claims, even if they did not directly espouse denialist positions. In Germany, on the other hand, the main far-right party, the AfD, provided organizational support to the anti-vax protests, and also helped in the spreading of conspiracy views among its electors, thus building upon their fears and mistrust. Aside from political allies, the convergence of a widespread New Age milieu with a strong Far Right was facilitated by visions of individual responsibility rather than collective solidarity on health issues, diffidence towards public intervention and proclaimed indifference towards social inequalities. Activists in both milieus also tried to exploit social fragmentation, which had been accentuated by the pandemic, addressing in particular those social groups that had been most penalized by the lockdown, especially from an economic point of view; all the more so in the eastern states where infection rates were initially lower. Additionally, the scapegoating of specific social groups (such as migrants and refugees) spread alongside the assumption of one's own superiority (in knowledge but also in immune defences). While these elements were also present in the other countries examined here, they found less support in Italy and remained extremely marginal in Greece.

More generally, the degree to which the anti-vax protests were politicized varied cross-nationally, being especially strong in contexts where populist right-wing leaders were in power and supported anti-vax protests in various ways. The most visible examples of this are the then presidents Jair Bolsonaro and Donald Trump, who have been prominent pandemic deniers and have openly opposed policies aimed at controlling the virus. In Brazil, Bolsonaro 'dismissed the virus as a "little cold" and blamed the media for "hysteria", suggesting that only a few thousand may die because of it' (Galanopoulos and Venizelos 2022: 7). In the United States, Trump had 'a history of expressing vaccine skepticism—including on the 2016 Republican debate stage—and sympathizing with prominent anti-vaccine advocates such as Robert Kennedy, Jr., who Trump had considered for a leadership role in a vaccine safety commission that ultimately never came to fruition'

(Snow and Bernatzky 2023: 189). Even during the initial phases of the pandemic, influential anti-vaccine organizations continued to be financed by the federal government.

It is also notable that far-right heads of state have often rejected the credibility of scientists and doctors through the mobilization of an alt-science network, in what have been defined as medical populist performances (Casarões and Magalhães 2021). Indeed, anti-vax positions were often used by far-right leaders in power (such as Donald Trump and Jair Bolsonaro, but also Narendra Modi and Benjamin Netanyahu) in order to mobilize consensus 'by empowering alt-science advocates and forging far-right transnational networks, … at the expense of mainstream science and national and international health authorities' (ibid.: 200).

Consequently, the degree to which positions relating to shelter in place orders, face masks, social distancing, and vaccination were politicized was particularly high in these countries. In the United States, the active support provided by Trump in opposition to vaccines and face masks, as well as his promotion of Covid-19 misinformation, contributed to politicizing vaccine resistance, which was more pronounced in Republican states than in those with a majority of Democratic Party supporters (Snow and Bernatzky 2023). High levels of politicization were also found in Brazil, where the anti-scientific rhetoric of Jair Bolsonaro encouraged his supporters to engage in incautious behaviour, after he 'minimized the risks of the disease, explicitly and publicly contradicting the instructions communicated by governors, the recommendations of the World Health Organization (WHO) and, more generally, the scientific community' (Ajzenman, Cavalcanti, and Da Mata 2020: 2).

Where far-right parties were in opposition, they also often (although not always) supported anti-vax protests and related conspiracy theories. While in states where governments adopted less stringent policies (such as in Sweden and the Netherlands), the Far Right pushed for stricter measures, in most countries far-right parties mobilized against what they (somewhat paradoxically) called 'authoritarian turns'. Therefore, in Spain the far-right Vox party embraced conspiracy arguments, including attacks on George Soros and accusations that the socialist party and Podemos coalitional governments were aiming 'to set up a communist regime' (FES Friedrich-Ebert-Stiftung 2021). In France, while not openly supporting anti-vax protests, Marine Le Pen denounced what she saw as a 'totalitarian-type lockdown', which she accused of ruining the country and being enacted 'under the fallacious pretext of public health', allowing the state to 'give permanent status to a large number of freedom-destroying measures' (ibid.).

In some countries, the Far Right also allied with the most conservative sections of the church in the spread of anti-vax conspiracy theories. Beyond the abovementioned Greek case, this can also be seen in Cyprus, where the National Popular Front (ELAM) shared the scepticism on mask-wearing and vaccination as well as the conspiratorial beliefs of its religious and nationalist base (ibid.) and in Romania, where the far-right Alliance for the Union of Romanians (AUR) coalesced with the Orthodox Church in supporting conspiracy beliefs and opposing the wearing of protective masks. In the United States, religious preachers in Evangelical sects supported the denialist positions of the Alt-Right, while in Southern Europe the same was true for small groupings in Catholic milieus.

Anti-vax protests: The short- and long-term effects on democracy

Although the anti-vax protests seem to have undergone a swift decline, following the reduced virulence of the virus and therefore the severity of anti-contagion measures, their actual and potential negative outcomes are not to be underestimated. Without claiming to offer a complete overview, I will now single out some of the vicious cycles and spirals that anti-vax protests seem to have triggered, thus transforming their environment in the short term, but also potentially in the long term.

First of all, at a micro level, a vicious cycle of increasing fear was triggered as anti-vax protests exploited existing anxieties and also contributed to strengthen them. This was especially the case with conspiracy theories, which spread terrorizing scenario among an already fearful constituency. Although short-term advantages can explain why some people turn to conspiracy theories, especially in uncertain times, belief in conspiracies is considered to be pathological in the long term, both for the individual and society as a whole. Factors that have been associated with adherence to conspiracy beliefs include paranoia, perceptions of a threat from societal change, uncertainty, powerlessness, and perceptions of lower social status. Generally speaking, conspiratorial impulses have been considered to represent 'agency panic', which triggered 'intense anxiety about an apparent loss of autonomy, the conviction that one's actions are being controlled by someone else, very often external agents' (Hellinger 2019: 6). Indeed, research has linked a strong proclivity toward conspiracy theories relating to immigrants, political dissidents, and a range of ethnic and religious groups to the insecurity fuelled by neoliberal developments, rather than simply to individual mental health issues (ibid.). During the Covid-19 pandemic, levels of fear increased with 'the sense of vulnerability triggered by the sustained threat to physical health, psychological well-being, and financial security. Uncertainty about the future is widespread. Expectations about everyday life have changed rapidly and dramatically, with top-down imposition of explanations and required responses, enforceable by law. Normal routines and plans have been thwarted' (Freeman et al. 2020: 2). This in turn led to a vicious cycle, in which uncertainty fuelled fears about powerful plots, with ensuing feelings of victimization and disempowerment for those who believed in them.

Another vicious cycle was linked to the politicized rejection of vaccination, which contributed to increased health hazards and infection rates among those who believed the fake news relating to the virus and vaccines, paving the way for new conspiratorial views (for instance, about the vaccinated spreading the virus and contributing to its mutation). Indeed, politicization can be seen to have had an impact on infection rates, as the spreading of conspiracy theories by far-right actors brought about reduced compliance with anti-contagion measures and therefore to the spread of the virus and related fears. The social danger caused by the diffusion of certain conspiracies has been considered to be particularly high during the pandemic, as it tended to reduce compliance with anti-contagion policies, including vaccination. In a number of countries, research has indicated that residents in provinces that lean towards extreme right-wing parties displayed lower rates of compliance with social distancing orders (Barbieri and Bonini 2020), with ensuing increases in infection rates. Even before the pandemic, research carried out in fourteen EU countries singled out a correlation between support for right-wing populist parties and a mistrust in vaccination (Kennedy 2019). The same phenomenon was confirmed in research that compared EU countries during the pandemic (Ivaldi and Mazzoleni 2021). In Germany, the presence of a higher number of Covid-19 deniers in a region was found to facilitate the spread of Covid-19, due to the fact that virus deniers were less likely to protect themselves against contagion, which also took place through participation in large gatherings in which anti-contagion measures were not respected (Lange and Monscheuer 2021).[1] Similarly, in the United States the perception of the risks related with Covid-19 were lower in counties with a high percentage of Trump voters (Barrios and Hochberg 2020), as Republican-controlled states

---

[1] Indeed, research indicated a strong correlation between electoral support for the AfD or other far-right parties and levels of Covid-19 contagion (Reuband 2021; Roose 2020). In addition, 'percentages for small parties of the far right as well as percentages of non-voters in the federal elections of 2005 and 2013 have positive effects on the progression of incidence, indicating a high persistence of political and democratic distance in parts of these regions' (Richter et al. 2021).

resisted social distancing policies (Charron, Lapuente, and Rodriguez-Pose 2022). Politicization tended to increase over time, resulting in higher and higher Covid-19 infection and fatality rates in pro-Trump counties, where local authorities' orders to shelter-in-place appeared to be less successful in encouraging physical distancing than in Democratic ones (Gollwitzer et al. 2020). These tendencies were strengthened by the consumption of conservative media (such as Fox News), which regularly downplayed the dangers of coronavirus (ibid.).[2]

Another spiralling effect is linked to the convergence in the anti-vax protests around conspiracy theories advanced by different actors on the Far Right, who could in turn also influence other actors in the net, including the New Age groupings. Indeed, the politicization of anti-vax positions is also reflected in the content of the conspiracy theories that have been espoused. Thus, conspiracies about Covid-19 in Germany were found to be particularly widespread among voters on the Right (at 28.0%), becoming gradually less common among voters for the Centre Right (17.3%) and the centre (14.7%), while only 8.8% of voters on the Left and 8.7% on the Centre Left expressed belief in such theories (Spöri and Eichhorn. 2021). In fact, as many as 54% of AfD supporters (compared to 20% of the overall population) believed that 'politicians and media consciously overstate the danger of Corona-Virus in order to cheat the public opinion'and that coronavirus is a 'pretext' to oppress the people (in the Autumn of 2020, this was true for 65% of AfD supporters compared to less than 14% of supporters of the CDU/CSU, SPD, Linken und Grünen (18% for the FDP supporters) (see Reuband 2021).[3] In addition to this, the politicization of the rejection of anti-contagion measures by the Far Right further increased the mistrust already widespread among its voters. To remain with the German example, the belief that Covid-19 is a conspiracy is linked to low levels of trust in government (25.6% versus 6.1%), as well as higher levels of trust in social media than in traditional media (43% compared to 7% of the entire population) (Spöri and Eichhorn 2021); and the same is also true for low levels of trust in science (Roozenbeek et al. 2020).[4]

---

[2] In the United States, it has been noted that during the pandemic, 'levels of politicization and polarization in newspaper coverage of COVID-19 meet or exceed levels found in coverage of global warming, which is one of the most polarizing issues in the public eye' (Hart, Chinn, and Soroka 2020).

[3] The spread of these beliefs among AfD supporters increased over time (up to 68% were against measures targeting the spread of Covid-19, even during the third wave), while they tended to decline in the rest of the population, where there was also increasing trust in official communication.

[4] In Saxony, areas with higher rates of infection from Covid-19 were often those with higher levels of electoral support for the AfD, where trust in the statements made by politicians concerning coronavirus were found to be lower (15% for AfD supporters against 44% in the wider population), and the same was true for trust in the public (29% vs. 45%), scientists (19% vs. 71%), and medical doctors (50% vs. 78%) (Wissenschaft im Dialog 2020: 48).

There is also a strong possibility that mistrust in science may spiral, as conspiracy theories provide for alternative 'truths'. In fact, 'The delegitimization of the medical establishment achieved by medical populists during the Covid-19 pandemic in many countries gained resonance precisely because of broad public mistrust of the medical and political establishments due to their connection with the profit-driven pharmaceutical industry, and their general inability to govern the crisis' (Bertuzzi, Lagalisse, Lello, Gobo, Sena 2022). Anti-vax conspiracy believers have been seen to testify to an increasing mistrust towards modern science that is linked to the spread of 'postmodern skepticism about "grand narratives", which has also led to a greater level of trust in complementary and alternative medicine in some parts of the population' (Harambam and Aupers 2015). Conspiracy theories have, in fact, been linked to specific critiques of science, such as 'the alleged dogmatism of modern science, the intimate relation of scientific knowledge production with vested interests, and the exclusion of lay knowledge by scientific experts forming a global "power elite"' (ibid.: 1). In this sense, it has been observed that 'More than merely mimicking modern science in order to augment epistemic authority, conspiracy theorists wish to purify it and reinstall its free spirit of inquiry. Their critique is targeted at the dogmatic nature of scientific assumptions, the authority of scientific institutions, and, indeed, the epistemic and social boundary work performed by scientists to sustain this authority. Science, we may say, is at once sacralized for its intentions but demonized for its manifestations' (ibid.). As a result of this, the vaccination controversy has been defined as addressing 'what it is to be a modern human, including questions about the responsibility one has to oneself, one's family and community, and the human community overall, as well as to the earth and its sustainability' (Hausman 2019, 32). This mistrust in science, however limited in size, could also have particularly serious effects on confidence in scientific expertise in the future.

Finally, a resilient effect can be singled out in the spread of authoritarian and anti-democratic political conceptions within regressive movements. Whereas protests on the Left often take the form of networked social movements, on the Right new groups emerged and others were transformed through the development of a plebiscitarian linkage between leaders and followers. As has so often occurred in the past, while the sources of discontent on the Left were framed within a discourse of solidarity and social justice, on the Right they were mostly placed within exclusive and xenophobic discourses within hierarchical organizational models. In their internal organizational structures, movements and parties on the Far Right build upon strong and personalized leadership rather than on citizen participation (della Porta et al.

2017), with appeals to the people coupled with hierarchical structures and exclusivist framing (Caiani and della Porta 2018). In general, while the participatory democracy proposed by progressive social movements points toward horizontal relations with an empowerment of the people, the populist vision put forward by right-wing actors 'does not require that mass constituencies engage in collective action at all, beyond the individual act of casting a ballot in national elections or popular referendums. Although both forms of popular subjectivity contest established elites, social movements mobilize such contestation from the bottom-up, whereas populism typically mobilizes mass constituencies from the top-down behind the leadership of a counter-elite' (Roberts 2015: 682). While there is undoubtedly also dissatisfaction on the Right with what is seen as an elitist trend, in this context the people are perceived in an exclusive and nativist form as the ethnos, rather than as the empowered citizens that we have seen as forming the basis of the visions of progressive movements.

The anti-vax mobilizations have the potential to broaden the Far Right's constituency, and with it its anti-democratic organizational models. While the strength of far-right actors has traditionally been interpreted as being linked to a fascist legacy (Taggart 1995), research on right-wing populism since the 2000s has especially pointed to the capacity of the Far Right to exploit new conflicts. Thus, 'Far-right collective actors are part of a large mobilization process by which they managed to politicise issues previously neglected by mainstream parties (e.g. immigration, minority issues, "law and order", welfare chauvinism; …). In this respect, the far right has been read through the lens of those economic and cultural grievances brought about by the process of globalization' (Castelli Gattinara and Pirro 2018: 7). The Great Recession at the beginning of the 2000s had already fuelled a Great Regression, which also revealed dynamics of competition on the regressive side, with the decline of the Centre Right (given its perceived lack of capacity to address economic and social crises) opening up spaces for parties on its right (Geiselberger 2017). Far-right movement organizations have, first and foremost, linked the socio-economic crisis to the opening of borders and the alleged threat that migrants pose to national identity (Wodak 2015), and in the wake of the Charlie Hebdo attacks have increasingly presented themselves as the defenders of Western values (della Porta et al. 2020).

Linked to transformation in the Far Right, the spread of conspiracies, which is increased by isolation, also triggers politically sectarian trends. Conspiracy thinking often brings about sectarian dynamics. As Lewis Coser (1954: 360) noted, 'A sect, as the Latin etymology suggests, consists of men who have cut themselves off from the main body of society. They have formed a restricted and closed group which rejects the norms of the inclusive society and proclaims its adherence to a special set of rules of conduct'. In his approach,

> The sect, by its exclusive structure, creates a morality opposed to that of the rest of society. Since it regards the outsider as not participating in grace, as not belonging to the select, as not yet having the fortitude or capacity to adhere to revolutionary principles, it sees him as an exponent of a lower morality … The sect requires the unreserved devotion of the individual to the rationale of the group. The exclusive group, being unable to avail itself of the advantage of large numbers, must attempt to offset it by the intensive exploitation of the loyalty of its members … Where the larger group can afford to leave its members leeway in opinions, attitudes and conduct, the sect must ever strive completely to subjugate the individual.
>
> **(ibid.)**

Our analysis has indicated just how much the frames and choreography of the anti-vax protests resonated with earlier anti-gender mobilizations. As they have inherited organizational fragmentation, victimization, scapegoating and fear from the anti-gender religious milieu, the anti-vax groupings have tended to retreat more and more into a parallel world in which defeat could be denied and one's own choices presented as heroic.

The risks posed by the abovementioned vicious cycles are all the more relevant given the amount of material resources that regressive movements have proven able to mobilize. While they have often been too easily considered as fuelled by the assumed conservatism of the working class, right-wing movements can instead be said to have a heterogeneous social background. As research on the political economy of the Far Right has pointed to, regressive movements are often sponsored by economic elites as well as by other components of what used to be considered the establishment. To give a few illustrations, the electoral campaigns of the Tea Party and Donald Trump in the US, and of far-right parties in Europe have all been generously financed by groups within the upper classes, which have also been pivotal in the construction of a global Far Right (Bob 2012). Moreover, the ultraconservative positions of the so-called 'anti-gender movements' have been sponsored by religious leaders—including the Vatican (Kuhar and Paternotte 2017)—as well as being helped by high levels of economic resources. It is from the split with the mainstream pro-life groups, oriented to more moderate and negotiated positions, that the anti-gender groups developed, considering the opposition to laity as non-negotiable aims, politicizing religion through strategies of lobbying of different parties as well as alliances with the Far Right. As Ayoub and Stoeckl (2023) noted, a politicized moral conservative network brings together 'actors that, at a first glance, have little in common: Russia, a series of Muslim states, as well as other states from Central and Eastern Europe and the Global South; Evangelicals and Orthodox Christians, Catholics, and Protestants; pro-life civil society groups and anti-migration right-wing populist parties, neoconservative media commentators, small businesses and homeowners, and entrepreneurs in the world of big business and economic consultancy'. Not by chance, the main international supporters of anti-gender actors, including Bolsonaro and Trump, also promoted anti-vax groupings.

This milieu has also found political and economic sponsors at an international level. While an entrepreneurial efforts made the QAnon conspiracy theory travel from the United States to Europe, research in the United States has pointed to the presence of a rich net of beneficiaries, which gains from the anti-vax positions and invests in strengthening them. Thus, in describing the anti-vax business, a civil society organization has pointed to the groups 'openly promoting lies and false cures' that 'comes from years of impunity in which they were hosted on popular social media platforms, driving traffic and advertising dollars to Facebook, Instagram, Twitter and YouTube, while benefiting from the enormous reach those platforms gladly afforded them' (Center for Countering Digital Hate 2021: 51). From an economic point of view, the report notes the presence of 'a dozen leading anti-vaxxers who operate businesses or organisations with significant revenues', being responsible for up to 70% of the anti-vaccine content shared on Facebook (half of which comes from Joseph Mercola, Del Bigtree, and Robert F. Kennedy Jr.)' (ibid.)[5]. Exactly how much money travelled to Europe and how this was achieved— as some of the twelve 'profiteers' singled out in the report were involved in doing—is an open question that must be dealt with by further research.

In summary, the pandemic has undoubtedly consolidated an 'unholy' alliance between the Far Right, ultraconservative religious fundamentalism and a New Age milieu, spreading conspiratorial visions to the broader anti-vax movement. It is not by chance that following the decline of the anti-vax protests, their channels of communication have often been involved in supporting not only Putin's Russia, but also anti-feminist and anti-gender as well as climate-change denialist positions. However, it is yet to be seen what the political and social effects of this priming of the anti-vaccination issue by the Far Right will be, especially given the fact that the world has already entered into another crisis caused by the impact on gas and oil prices of the war in Ukraine and the related sanctions with the climate crisis in full speed.

---

[5] With more than $1.5 million in federal loans through the program designed to help businesses through the Covid pandemic and annual revenues of about $36 millions, 22 antivax organizations employ 266 people (ibid.).

References

Ajzenman, Nicolas, Tiago Cavalcanti, and Daniel Da Mata. 2020. 'More Than Words: Leaders' Speech and Risky Behavior during a Pandemic'. SSRN Scholarly Paper. Rochester, NY. https://doi.org/10.2139/ssrn.3582908.

Aldred, Lisa. 2000. 'Plastic Shamans and Astroturf Sun Dances: New Age Commercialization of Native American Spirituality'. *American Indian Quarterly* 24 (3): 329–52.

Allen, Amy. 2016. *The End of Progress: Decolonizing the Normative Foundations of Critical Theory*. New York: Columbia University Press.

Alter, Karen, J., and Michael Zürn. 2020. 'Theorising Backlash Politics: Conclusion to a Special Issue on Backlash Politics in Comparison'. *The British Journal of Politics and International Relations* 22 (4): 739–52.

Alteri, Luca, Louisa Parks, Luca Raffini, and Tommaso Vitale. 2021. 'Covid-19 and the Structural Crisis of Liberal Democracies. Determinants and Consequences of the Governance of Pandemic'. *Partecipazione e Conflitto* 14 (1): 1–37.

Anello, Paola, Laura Cestari, Tatjana Baldovin, Lorenzo Simonato, Gabriella Frasca, Nicola Caranci, Maria Grazia Pascucci, Francesca Valent, and Cristina Canova. 2017. 'Socioeconomic Factors Influencing Childhood Vaccination in Two Northern Italian Regions'. *Vaccine* 35 (36): 4673–80. https://doi.org/10.1016/j.vaccine.2017.07.058.

Asprem, Egil, and Asbjørn Dyrendal. 2015. 'Conspirituality Reconsidered: How Surprising and How New is the Confluence of Spirituality and Conspiracy Theory?' *Journal of Contemporary Religion* 30 (3): 367–82. https://doi.org/10.1080/13537903.2015.1081339.

Ayoub, Phillip, M., and Kristina Stoeckl. 2023. *Global Resistances to LGBTI Rights: Actors, Venues of Contestation*. New York: NYU Press.

Azmanova, Albena. 2021. 'Battlegrounds of Justice: The Pandemic and What Really Grieves the 99%'. In *Pandemics, Politics and Society: Critical Perspectives on the Covid-19 Crisis*, edited by Gerard Delanty, 243–55. Berlin: De Gruyter.

Balandat, Felix, Nikolai Schreiter, and Annette Seidel-Arpaci. 2021. 'Antisemitismus Als Zentrales Ideologieelement Bei Den Coronaprotesten'. In *Fehlender Mindestabstand. Die Coronakrise Und Die Netzwerke Der Demokratiefeinde*, edited by Kleffner Heike and Matthias Meisner, 102–8. Freiburg: Herder.

Baldwin, Peter. 2005. *Disease and Democracy: The Industrialized World Faces AIDS*. Berkeley: University of California Press.

Barbieri, Paolo, and Beatrice Bonini. 2020. 'Political Orientation and Adherence to Social Distancing During the COVID-19 Pandemic in Italy'. SSRN Scholarly Paper. Rochester, NY. https://doi.org/10.2139/ssrn.3640324.

Bargain, Olivier, and Ulugbek Aminjonov. 2020. *Trust and Compliance to Public Health Policies in Times of COVID-19*. Bonn: IZA Institute of Labor Economics. https://docs.iza.org/dp13205.pdf.

Barkun, Michael. 2013. *A Culture of Conspiracy: Apocalyptic Visions in Contemporary America*. 2nd edition. Berkeley: University of California Press.

Barrios, John M and Yael Hochberg. 2020. Risk Perception Through the Lens of Politics in the Time of the COVID-19 Pandemic. National Bureau of Economic Research Working Paper Series No 27008. https://doi.org/10.3386/w27008.

Bauman, Zygmunt. 1997. *Postmodernity and Its Discontents*. Cambridge: Polity.

————. 2000. *Liquid Modernity*. Oxford: Polity.

Beissinger, Mark R. 2002. *Nationalist Mobilization and the Collapse of the Soviet State*. Cambridge Studies in Comparative Politics. Cambridge: Cambridge University Press. https://doi.org/10.1017/CBO9780511613593.

Benford, Robert D., and David A. Snow. 2000. 'Framing Processes and Social Movements: An Overview and Assessment'. *Annual Review of Sociology* 26: 611–39.

Bennett, W. Lance, and Alexandra Segerberg. 2013. *The Logic of Connective Action: Digital Media and the Personalization of Contentious Politics*. Cambridge Studies in Contentious Politics. Cambridge: Cambridge University Press. https://doi.org/10.1017/CBO9781139198752.

Benz, Wolfgang, ed. 2021a. *Querdenken. Protestbewegung Zwischen Demokratieverachtung, Hass und Aufruhr*. Berlin: Metropol Verlag.

————. 2021b. 'Warum Sind Verschwörungsmythen so Attraktiv?' In *Querdenken. Protestbewegung Zwischen Demokratieverachtung, Hass und Aufruhr*, edited by Wolfgang Benz, 76–99. Berlin: Metropol Verlag.

Berezin, Mabel. 2009. *Illiberal Politics in Neoliberal Times: Culture, Security and Populism in the New Europe*. Cambridge: Cambridge University Press. https://cadmus.eui.eu/handle/1814/10968.

Bertuzzi, Niccolò, Erica Lagalisse, Elisa Lello, Giampietro Gobo and Barbara Sena. 2022. 'Politics during and after Covid-19: Science, Health and Social Protest'. *Partecipazione e Conflitto* [Online] 15 (3): 507–29.

Bianchetti, Federico. 2022. 'Un prof di Milano occupa la scuola contro la Dad per gli studenti non vaccinati'. Skuola.net—Portale per Studenti: Materiali, Appunti e Notizie (blog). 4 February 2022. https://www.skuola.net/scuola/prof-milano-occupa-scuola-contro-dad-non-vaccinati.html.

Bicchieri, Cristina, Eugen Dimant, Simon Gaechter, and Daniele Nosenzo. 2020. 'Observability, Social Proximity, and the Erosion of Norm Compliance'. SSRN Scholarly Paper. Rochester, NY. https://doi.org/10.2139/ssrn.3576289.

Bob, Clifford. 2012. *The Global Right Wing and the Clash of World Politics*. Cambridge Studies in Contentious Politics. Cambridge: Cambridge University Press. https://doi.org/10.1017/CBO9781139031042.

Bobbio, Norberto. 1997. 'Revolution Between Movement and Change'. *Thesis Eleven* 48: 113–29. https://doi.org/10.1177/0725513697048000008.

Boberg, Svenja, Thorsten Quandt, Tim Schatto-Eckrodt, and Lena Frischlich. 2020. 'Pandemic Populism: Facebook Pages of Alternative News Media and the Corona Crisis—A Computational Content Analysis'. Muenster Online Research (MOR) Working Paper 1/2020. arXiv. http://arxiv.org/abs/2004.02566.

Bracewell, Lorna. 2021. 'Gender, Populism, and the QAnon Conspiracy Movement'. *Frontiers in Sociology* 5: 615727. https://doi.org/10.3389/fsoc.2020.615727.

Bracke, Sarah, Wannes Dupont, and David Paternotte. 2017. '"No Prophet Is Accepted in His Own Country": Catholic Anti-Gender Activism in Belgium'. In *Anti-Gender Campaigns in Europe: Mobilising against Equality*, edited by Roman Kuhar and David Paternotte, 41–58. London: Rowman & Littlefield International.

Bringel, B, and G Pleyers. 2020. 'Introducion: La Pandemia y El Suo Eco Global'. In *Alerta Global*, edited by B. Bringel and G. Pleyers, 9–33. Buenos Aires: Clacso.

Brodeur, Abel, Idaliya Grigoryeva, and Lamis Kattan. 2021. 'Stay-at-Home Orders, Social Distancing, and Trust'. *Journal of Population Economics* 34 (4): 1321–54. https://doi.org/10.1007/s00148-021-00848-z.

Brown, Susan Love. 1992. 'Baby Boomers, American Character, and the New Age: A Synthesis'. In *Perspectives on the New Age*, edited by J. R. Lewis and J. G. Melton, 87–96. Albany:

State University of New York Press. https://sunypress.edu/Books/P/Perspectives-on-the-New-Age.

Brubaker, Rogers. 2020. 'Populism and Nationalism'. *Nations and Nationalism* 26 (1): 44–66. https://doi.org/10.1111/nana.12522.

Butter, Michael. 2021. *»Nichts Ist, Wie Es Scheint« Über Verschwörungstheorien.* Berlin: Suhrkamp.

Caiani, Manuela, and Donatella della Porta. 2018. 'The Radical Right as Social Movement Organizations'. In *The Oxford Handbook on the Radical Right*, edited by Jens Rydgren, 327–47. Oxford: Oxford University Press.

Caiani, Manuela, Donatella della Porta, and Claudius Wagemann. 2012. *Mobilizing on the Extreme Right: Germany, Italy, and the United States.* Oxford: Oxford University Press. https://cadmus.eui.eu/handle/1814/20555.

Casarões, Guilherme, and David Magalhães. 2021. 'The Hydroxychloroquine Alliance: How Far-Right Leaders and Alt-Science Preachers Came Together to Promote a Miracle Drug'. *Revista de Administração Pública* 55 (March): 197–214. https://doi.org/10.1590/0034-761220200556.

Castelli Gattinara, Pietro, and Andrea L. P. Pirro. 2018. 'The Far Right as Social Movement'. *European Societies* 21 (4): 447–62. https://doi.org/10.1080/14616696.2018.1494301.

Center for Countering Digital Hate. 2021. 'Pandemic Profiteers: The Business of Anti-Vaxx'. https://counterhate.com/wp-content/uploads/2022/05/210601-Pandemic-Profiteers-Report.pdf.

Charron, Nicholas, Victor Lapuente and Andrés Rodríguez-Pose. 2022 "Uncooperative society, uncooperative politics or both? Trust, polarization, populism and COVID-19 deaths across European regions." *European Journal of Political Research* (online preprint)

Christou, Stella. 2022. 'Collective Reactions to COVID-19 Containment Measures in Greece: Mapping the Greek Anti-Vax and Beyond'. Internal Report. Florence: Scuola Normale Superiore.

Clemens, Elisabeth, S., and Debra Minkoff C. 2004. 'Beyond the Iron Law: Rethinking the Place of Organizations in Social Movement Research'. In *The Blackwell Companion to Social Movements*, edited by David A. Snow, Sarah Soule A., and Hanspeter Kriesi, 156–70. New Jersey: Blackwell Publishing Ltd.

Cofrancesco, Dino. 1981. *Destra e sinistra.* Genoa: Il Basilisco.

Collier, David, and Gerardo L. Munck. 2017. 'Building Blocks and Methodological Challenges: A Framework for Studying Critical Junctures'. SSRN Scholarly Paper. Rochester, NY. https://papers.ssrn.com/abstract=3034920.

Coser, Lewis A. 1954. *Toward a sociology of social conflict.* PhD Thesis. ProQuest Dissertations and Theses. Columbia University. 302005883. https://www.proquest.com/dissertations-theses/toward-sociology-social-conflict/docview/302005883/se-2?accountid=12830.

Crossley, Nick. 2006. *Contesting Psychiatry: Social Movements in Mental Health.* Routledge.

'Crowdsourcing'. 2022. In *Wikipedia.* https://en.wikipedia.org/w/index.php?title=Crowdsourcing&oldid=1128372694.

De Sousa Santos, Boaventura. 2020. 'El Coronavirus y Nuestra Contemporaneidad'. In *Alerta Global*, edited by B. Bringel and G. Pleyers, 35–40. Buenos Aires: Clacso.

Delanty, Gerard. 2021. *Pandemics, Politics, and Society: Critical Perspectives on the Covid-19 Crisis.* Berlin: De Gruyter. https://doi.org/10.1515/9783110713350.

della Porta, Donatella. 1995. *Social Movements, Political Violence, and the State: A Comparative Analysis of Italy and Germany.* Cambridge: Cambridge University Press.

———. 2009. 'Democracy in Movement: Some Conclusions'. In *Democracy in Social Movements*, edited by Donatella della Porta, 262–74. London: Palgrave Macmillan UK. https://doi.org/10.1057/9780230240865_12.

———. 2013. *Can Democracy Be Saved? Participation, Deliberation and Social Movements*. New Jersey: John Wiley & Sons.

———. 2015. *Social Movements in Times of Austerity: Bringing Capitalism Back into Protest Analysis*. Cambridge, MA: Polity.

———. 2019. 'Deconstructing Generations in Movements: Introduction'. *American Behavioral Scientist* 63 (10): 1407–26. https://doi.org/10.1177/0002764219831739.

———. 2020. 'How Progressive Social Movements Can Save Democracy in Pandemic Times'. *Interface: A Journal for and about Social Movements* 12 (1): 355–58.

———. 2022. *Contentious Politics in Emergency Critical Junctures: Progressive Social Movements during the Pandemic*. Elements in Contentious Politics. Cambridge: Cambridge University Press.

della Porta, Donatella, Massimiliano Andretta, Tiago Fernandes, Eduardo Romanos, Francis Patrick O'Connor, and Markos Vogiatzoglou. 2017. *Late Neoliberalism and Its Discontents in the Economic Crisis: Comparing Social Movements in the European Periphery*. Cham: Palgrave Macmillan. https://doi.org/10.1007/978-3-319-35080-6.

della Porta, Donatella, Niccolò Bertuzzi, Daniela Chironi, Chiara Milan, Martín Portos, and Lorenzo Zamponi. 2022. *Resisting the Backlash: Street Protest in Italy*. London: Routledge. https://doi.org/10.4324/9781003262558.

della Porta, Donatella, and Mario Diani. 2020. *Social Movements: An Introduction*. 3rd edition. New Jersey: Wiley-Blackwell.

della Porta, Donatella, Pietro Castelli Gattinara, Konstantinos Eleftheriadis, and Andrea Felicetti. 2020. *Discursive Turns and Critical Junctures: Debating Citizenship after the Charlie Hebdo Attacks*. Oxford: Oxford University Press. https://doi.org/10.1093/oso/9780190097431.001.0001.

della Porta, Donatella, Hans Jonas Gunzelmann, and Martín Portos. 2021. 'Repression and Democracy Amidst the Eventful 1-O Referendum'. In *Catalan Independence and the Crisis of Sovereignty*, edited by Óscar García Agustín, 127–50. Cham: Springer International Publishing. https://doi.org/10.1007/978-3-030-54867-4_6.

della Porta, Donatella, Sophia Hunger, Swen Hutter, and Anna Lavizzari. (forthcoming). 'Expanding Protest Event Analysis through Videos'. Internal Report.

della Porta, Donatella, and Anna Lavizzari. 2022. 'Waves in Cycle: The Protests against Anti-contagion Measures and Vaccination in Covid-19 times in Italy'. *Partecipazione e Conflitto* [Online] 15 (3): 720–40.

della Porta, Donatella, and Alice Mattoni, eds. 2014. *Spreading Protest. Social Movements in Times of Crisis*. Essex: ECPR Press. https://opac.units.it/sebina/repository/catalogazione/immagini/PDF/spreading%20protest.pdf.

della Porta, Donatella, and Dieter Rucht. 1995. 'Left-Libertarian Movements in Context: A Comparison of Italy and West Germany, 1965–1990'. In *The Politics of Social Protest: Comparative Perspectives on States and Social Movements*, edited by J. Craig Jenkins and Bert Klandermans, 229–72. Minneapolis: University of Minnesota Press. http://www.jstor.org/stable/10.5749/j.ctttt723.11.

della Porta, Donatella, and Sidney Tarrow. 1986. 'Unwanted Children: Political Violence and the Cycle of Protest in Italy, 1966–1973'. *European Journal of Political Research* 14 (5–6): 607–32. https://doi.org/10.1111/j.1475-6765.1986.tb00852.x.

Drazkiewitz, Elżbieta. 2022. 'Virtuosos of Mimesis and Mimicry: A Case Study of Movements Propagating Conspiracy Theories in Ireland and Poland'. *Partecipazione e Conflitto* [Online] 15 (3): 651–71.

Eatwell, Roger. 1996. *Fascism: A History*. 1st American ed. New York: Allen Lane.

Eisenmann, Clemens, Sebastian Koch, and Christian Meyer. 2021. 'Rhetoriken Skeptischer Vergemeinschaftung'. In *Die Misstrauensgemeinschaft Der »Querdenker«: Die*

Corona-Proteste Aus Kultur- Und Sozialwissenschaftlicher Perspektive, edited by Sven Reichardt, 185–224. Frankfurt: Campus Verlag.

Eyal, Gil. 2019. *The Crisis of Expertise*. Cambridge: Polity.

European Parliament. 2020. 'States of Emergency in Response to the Coronavirus Crisis: Normative Response and Parliamentary Oversight in the EU Member States during the First Wave of the Pandemic'. LU: European Parliament. https://data.europa.eu/doi/10.2861/892605.

Farjam, Mike, Federico Bianchi, Flaminio Squazzoni, and Giangiacomo Bravo. 2021. 'Dangerous Liaisons: An Online Experiment on the Role of Scientific Experts and Politicians in Ensuring Public Support for Anti-COVID Measures'. *Royal Society Open Science* 8 (3): 201310. https://doi.org/10.1098/rsos.201310.

Fassin, Didier. 2021. 'Of Plots and Men: The Heuristics of Conspiracy Theories'. *Current Anthropology* 62 (2): 128–37.

FES Friedrich-Ebert-Stiftung. 2021. 'The Profiteers of Fear? Right-Wing Populism and the COVID-19 Crisis'. FES Friedrich-Ebert-Stiftung. https://nordics.fes.de/e/default-7f5ab95431.

Fillieule, Olivier, and Manuel Jiménez. 2003. 'The Methodology of Protest Event Analysis and the Media Politics of Reporting Environmental Protest Events'. In *Environmental Protest in Western Europe*, edited by Christopher Rootes, 258–79. Oxford: Oxford University Press. https://doi.org/10.1093/0199252068.005.0001.

Flesher Fominaya, Cristina. 2021. 'Mobilizing During the Covid-19 Pandemic: From Democratic Innovation to The Political Weaponization of Disinformation'. *OSF Preprints*. d3pke. Center for Open Science. https://ideas.repec.org//p/osf/osfxxx/d3pke.html.

Fligstein, Neil, and Doug McAdam. 2012. *A Theory of Fields*. Oxford: Oxford University Press.

Frazzetta, Federica. 2022. *L' Onda Nera Frastagliata. L'estrema Destra Nell'Italia Del Nuovo Millennio*. Milano: Meltemi.

Freeman, Daniel, Felicity Waite, Laina Rosebrock, Ariane Petit, Chiara Causier, Anna East, Lucy Jenner, et al. 2020. 'Coronavirus Conspiracy Beliefs, Mistrust, and Compliance with Government Guidelines in England'. *Psychological Medicine* 52 (2): 251–63. https://doi.org/:10.1017/S0033291720001890.

Frei, Nadine, and Oliver Nachtwey. 2021. *Quellen des «Querdenkertums». Eine politische Soziologie der Corona-Proteste in Baden-Württemberg* Preprint. Basel: Fachbereich Soziologie, Universität Basel. https://doi.org/10.31235/osf.io/8f4pb.

Froio, Caterina. 2018. 'Race, Religion, or Culture? Framing Islam between Racism and Neo-Racism in the Online Network of the French Far Right'. *Perspectives on Politics* 16 (3): 696–709. https://doi.org/10.1017/S1537592718001573.

Galanopoulos, Antonis, and Giorgos Venizelos. 2022. 'Anti-Populism and Populist Hype During the COVID-19 Pandemic'. *Representation* 58 (2): 251–68. https://doi.org/10.1080/00344893.2021.2017334.

Gamson, William A. 2013. 'Injustice Frames'. In *The Wiley-Blackwell Encyclopedia of Social and Political Movements*, edited by David A. Snow, Donatella della Porta, Bert Klandermans and Doug McAdam, 607–8. Malden: Wiley-Blackwell John Wiley & Sons, Ltd. https://doi.org/10.1002/9780470674871.wbespm110.

Gamson, William A., Bruce Fireman, and Steven Rytina. 1982. *Encounters with Unjust Authority*. Illinois: The Dorsey Press.

García Agustín, Óscar, and Anita Nissen. 2022. 'The Anti-Restrictions Movement and the Populist Counterpublics in Denmark'. *Partecipazione e Conflitto* [Online], 15 (3): 741–60.

Geiselberger, Heinrich. 2017. *The Great Regression*. Cambridge: Polity. https://www.wiley.com/en-br/The+Great+Regression-p-9781509522361.

Gerbaudo, Paolo. 2020. 'The Pandemic Crowd: Protest in the Time of Covid-19'. *Journal of International Affairs* 73 (2): 61–76.

Gerlach, Luther P., and Virginia H. Hine. 1970. *People, Power, Change; Movements of Social Transformation*. Indianapolis: Bobbs-Merrill.

Gesser-Edelsburg, Anat, Yaffa Shir-Raz, and Manfred S. Green. 2016. 'Why Do Parents Who Usually Vaccinate Their Children Hesitate or Refuse? General Good vs. Individual Risk'. *Journal of Risk Research* 19 (4): 405–24. https://doi.org/10.1080/13669877.2014.983947.

Gollwitzer, Anton, Cameron Martel, William J. Brady, Philip Pärnamets, Isaac G. Freedman, Eric D. Knowles, and Jay J. Van Bavel. 2020. 'Partisan Differences in Physical Distancing Are Linked to Health Outcomes during the COVID-19 Pandemic'. *Nature Human Behaviour* 4 (11): 1186–97. https://doi.org/10.1038/s41562-020-00977-7.

Goyal, Nihit, and Michael Howlett. 2021. '"Measuring the Mix" of Policy Responses to COVID-19: Comparative Policy Analysis Using Topic Modelling'. *Journal of Comparative Policy Analysis: Research and Practice* 23 (2): 250–61. https://doi.org/10.1080/13876988.2021.1880872.

Grignolio, Andrea. 2016. *Chi ha paura dei vaccini?* Torino: Codice Edizioni.

Hammer, Olav. 2001. *Claiming Knowledge: Strategies of Epistemology from Theosophy to the New Age*. Köln: E. J. Brill.

———. 2006. 'New Age Movement'. In *Dictionary of Gnosis and Western Esotericism*, edited by Wouter J. Hanegraaff, 855–61. Leiden: E.J. Brill.

Hanegraaff, Wouter J. 1996. *New Age Religion and Western Culture: Esotericism in the Mirror of Secular Thought*. Leiden: E.J. Brill. https://sunypress.edu/Books/N/New-Age-Religion-and-Western-Culture.

Hanloser, Gerhard. 2021. '"Nicht rechts, nicht links"? Ideologien und Aktionsformen der "Corona-Rebellen"'. *Sozial Geschichte Online*, 43.

Hannah, Matthew N. 2021. 'A Conspiracy of Data: QAnon, Social Media, and Information Visualization'. *Social Media + Society* 7.

Harambam, Jaron, and Stef Aupers. 2015. 'Contesting Epistemic Authority: Conspiracy Theories on the Boundaries of Science'. *Public Understanding of Science* 24 (4): 466–80. https://doi.org/10.1177/0963662514559891.

Harsin, Jayson. 2020. 'Toxic White Masculinity, Post-Truth Politics and the COVID-19 Infodemic'. *European Journal of Cultural Studies* 23 (6): 1060–68. https://doi.org/10.1177/1367549420944934.

Hausman, Bernice L. 2019. *Anti/Vax*. New York: Cornell University Press. http://www.jstor.org/stable/10.7591/j.ctvdtphd8.

Heelas, Paul. 1996. *The New Age Movement: Religion, Culture and Society in the Age of Postmodernity*. Cambridge: Blackwell Publishing Ltd.

———. 2006. 'Nursing Spirituality'. *Spirituality and Health International* 7 (1): 8–23. https://doi.org/10.1002/shi.64.

Heelas, Paul, and Linda Woodhead. 2005. *The Spiritual Revolution: Why Religion Is Giving Way to Spirituality*. Walden MA: Blackwell.

Hellinger, Daniel C. 2019. *Conspiracies and Conspiracy Theories in the Age of Trump*. Cham: Springer International Publishing. https://doi.org/10.1007/978-3-319-98158-1.

Holzer, Boris. 2021. 'Zwischen Protest und Parodie: Strukturen der »Querdenken«-Kommunikation auf Telegram (und anderswo)'. In *Die Misstrauensgemeinschaft der »Querdenker«: Die Corona-Proteste aus kultur- und sozialwissenschaftlicher Perspektive*, edited by Sven Reichardt, 125–57. Frankfurt: Campus Verlag. https://doi.org/10.31235/osf.io/9rgtk.

Horton, Richard. 2020. 'Offline: COVID-19 Is Not a Pandemic'. *The Lancet* 396 (10255): 874. https://doi.org/10.1016/S0140-6736(20)32000-6.

Hoseini, Mohamad, Philipe Melo, Fabricio Benevenuto, Anja Feldmann, and Savvas Zannettou. 2021. 'On the Globalization of the QAnon Conspiracy Theory Through Telegram'. In

Proceedings of the ACM on Human-Computer Interaction 5, 1–24. https://doi.org/10.48550/arXiv.2105.13020.

Hunger, Sophia, Eylem Kanol, Daniel Saldivia Gonzatti, and Swen Hutter. 2021. 'Breeding Grounds for Radicalization? Regional Determinants of Anti-System Protest in Germany'. Center of Civil Society Research Working Paper 2021. WZB: Berlin.

Hutter, Swen. 2014. *Protesting Culture and Economics in Western Europe.* Minneapolis: University of Minnesota Press. https://www.upress.umn.edu/book-division/books/protesting-culture-and-economics-in-western-europe.

International Institute for Democracy and Electoral Assistance (International IDEA). 2021a. *Electoral Processes: Navigating and Emerging from Crisis (Global State of Democracy Thematic Paper 2021).* https://doi.org/10.31752/idea.2021.85.

———. 2021b. *The State of Democracy in Europe 2021: Overcoming the Impact of the Pandemic.* https://doi.org/10.31752/idea.2021.96.

Ivaldi, Gilles, and Oscar Mazzoleni. 2021. 'Linking Covid-19-Related Socio-Economic Anxieties with Right-Wing Populism: A Comparison between Europe and the United States'. ECPR General Conference Working paper 2021. ECPR: Innsbruck. https://shs.hal.science/halshs-03335324.

Jasper, James M., and Jan Willem Duyvendak, eds. 2015. *Players and Arenas: The Interactive Dynamics of Protest.* Amsterdam: Amsterdam University Press. https://www.jstor.org/stable/j.ctt16vj285.

Johnston, Hank. 2018. 'The Revenge of Turner and Killian: Paradigm, State, and Repertoire in Social Movement Research'. COSMOS May 26–28 Conference Paper. Florence: Scuola Normale Superiore.

Johnston, Hank, and Bert Klandermans, eds. 1995. *Social Movements and Culture.* 1st edition. Minneapolis: University of Minnesota Press.

Juris, Jeffrey S. 2012. 'Reflections on #Occupy Everywhere: Social Media, Public Space, and Emerging Logics of Aggregation'. *American Ethnologist* 39 (2): 259–79. https://doi.org/10.1111/j.1548-1425.2012.01362.x.

Kallis, Giorgos, Susan Paulson, Giacomo D'Alisa and Federico Demaria. 2020. *The case for degrowth.* Cambridge, UK: Polity Press.

Kanter, Rosabeth Moss. 1968. 'Commitment and Social Organization: A Study of Commitment Mechanisms in Utopian Communities'. *American Sociological Review* 33: 499–517. https://doi.org/10.2307/2092438.

———. 1972. *Commitment and Community: Communes and Utopias in Sociological Perspective.* Cambridge, MA: Harvard University Press.

Kennedy, Jonathan. 2019. 'Populist Politics and Vaccine Hesitancy in Western Europe: An Analysis of National-Level Data'. *European Journal of Public Health* 29 (3): 512–6. https://doi.org/10.1093/eurpub/ckz004.

Kitschelt, Herbert. 1995. 'Formation of Party Cleavages in Post-Communist Democracies: Theoretical Propositions'. *Party Politics* 1 (4): 447–72. https://doi.org/10.1177/1354068895001004002.

Klandermans, Bert. 2013. 'Motivation and Types of Motives (Instrumental; Identity, Ideological Motives)'. In *The Wiley-Blackwell Encyclopedia of Social and Political Movements*, edited by David A. Snow, Donatella della Porta, Bert Klandermans, and Doug McAdam, 778–80. Malden: Wiley-Blackwell John Wiley & Sons, Ltd. https://doi.org/10.1002/9780470674871.wbespm133.

Kleffner, Heike, and Mattias Meisner, eds. 2021. *Fehlender Mindestabstand Die Coronakrise und die Netzwerke der Demokratiefeinde.* Freiburg: Herder. https://www.herder.de/geschichte-politik/shop/p4/71056-fehlender-mindestabstand-klappenbroschur/.

Kleres, Jochen. 2018. *The Social Organization of Disease: Emotions and Civic Action.* London: Routledge. https://doi.org/10.4324/9781315708812.

Koopmans, Ruud. 2004. 'Movements and Media: Selection Processes and Evolutionary Dynamics in the Public Sphere'. *Theory and Society* 33 (3): 367–91. https://doi.org/10.1023/B:RYSO.0000038603.34963.de.

Koopmans, Ruud, and Dieter Rucht. 2002. 'Protest Event Analysis'. In *Methods of Social Movement Research*, edited by Bert Klandermans and Suzanne Staggenborg, 213–59. Minneapolis: University of Minnesota Press.

Koos, Sebastian. 2021. 'Konturen einer heterogenen »Misstrauensgemeinschaft«: Die soziale Zusammensetzung der Corona-Proteste und die Motive ihrer Teilnehmer:innen'. In *Die Misstrauensgemeinschaft der »Querdenker«: Die Corona-Proteste aus kultur- und sozialwissenschaftlicher Perspektive*, edited by Sven Reichardt, 67–90. Frankfurt: Campus Verlag. https://kops.uni-konstanz.de/handle/123456789/54272.

Kreuder-Sonnen, Christian. 2019. *Emergency Powers of International Organizations: Between Normalization and Containment*. Oxford: Oxford University Press.

Kriesi, Hanspeter, Ruud Koopmans, Jain Willem Duyvendak, and Marco Giugni. 1995. *New Social Movements in Western Europe: A Comparative Analysis*. Minneapolis: University of Minnesota Press. https://archive-ouverte.unige.ch/unige:92400.

Kuhar, Roman, and David Paternotte. 2017. *Anti-Gender Campaigns in Europe: Mobilising against Equality*. London: Rowman & Littlefield International.

Lange, Martin, and Ole Monscheuer. 2021. 'Spreading the Disease: Protest in Times of Pandemics'. ZEW Discussion Papers 21–009. ZEW—Leibniz Centre for European Economic Research. https://ideas.repec.org/p/zbw/zewdip/21009.html.

Laponce, Jean A. 1981. *Left and Right: The Topography of Political Perceptions*. Toronto: University of Toronto press.

Lavizzari, Anna. 2021. *Protesting Gender: The LGBTIQ Movement and Its Opponents in Italy*. Oxford, UK: Routledge.

Lavizzari, Anna, and Massimo Prearo. 2019. 'The Anti-Gender Movement in Italy: Catholic Participation between Electoral and Protest Politics'. *European Societies* 21 (3): 422–42. https://doi.org/10.1080/14616696.2018.1536801.

Lello, Elisa. 2020. 'Populismo Anti-Scientifico o Nodi Irrisolti Della Biomedicina? Prospettive a Confronto Intorno al Movimento Free Vax'. *Rassegna Italiana Di Sociologia*, no. 3/2020. https://doi.org/10.1423/98558.

Lello, Elisa, Niccolò Bertuzzi, Marco Pedroni, and Luca Raffini. 2022. 'Vaccine hesitancy and refusal during the Covid-19 pandemic in Italy: Individualistic claims or repoliticization?' *Partecipazione e Conflitto* [Online], 15 (30): 672–96.

Lindekilde, Lasse. 2014. 'Discourse and Frame Analysis'. In *Methodological Practices in Social Movement Research*, edited by Donatella della Porta, 195–227. Oxford: Oxford University Press. https://doi.org/10.1093/acprof:oso/9780198719571.003.0009.

Lofland, John. 1985. *Protest: Studies of Collective Behaviour and Social Movements*. Oxford, UK: Routledge. https://www.routledge.com/Protest-Studies-of-Collective-Behaviour-and-Social-Movements/Lofland/p/book/9780887388767.

———. 1995. 'Charting Degrees of Movement Culture: Tasks of the Cultural Cartograph'. In *Social Movements and Culture*, edited by Hank Johnston and Bert Klandermans, 1st edition, 250–75. Minneapolis: University of Minnesota Press.

MacKian, Sara. 2012. *Everyday Spirituality: Social and Spatial Worlds of Enchantment*. Basingstoke, UK: Palgrave Macmillan.

Mancosu, Moreno, Salvatore Vassallo, and Cristiano Vezzoni. 2017. 'Believing in Conspiracy Theories: Evidence from an Exploratory Analysis of Italian Survey Data'. *South European Society and Politics* 22 (3): 327–44. https://doi.org/10.1080/13608746.2017.1359894.

Mayer, Stefanie, and Birgit Sauer. 2017. '"Gender Ideology" in Austria: Coalitions around an Empty Signifier'. In *Anti-Gender Campaigns in Europe: Mobilising against Equality*, edited by Roman Kuhar and David Paternotte, 23–40. London: Rowman & Littlefield International.

McCarthy, John D., Clark McPhail, and Jackie Smith. 1996. 'Images of Protest: Dimensions of Selection Bias in Media Coverage of Washington Demonstrations, 1982 and 1991'. *American Sociological Review* 61 (3): 478–99. https://doi.org/10.2307/2096360.

McNeill, William. 1977. *Plagues and Peoples*. New York: Anchor.

Melucci, Alberto. 1990. *1990 Sistema Politico, Partiti e Movimenti Sociali*. Milano: Feltrineli.

Minkenberg, Michael. 2011. *The Radical Right in Europe: An Overview*. Gütersloh: Bertelsmann Stiftung. https://www.bertelsmann-stiftung.de/en/publications/publication/did/the-radical-right-in-europe-an-overview.

Morsello, Barbara, and Paolo Giardullo. 2022. 'Free Choice in the Making: Vaccine-related Activism as an Alternative form of Citizenship during the Covid-19 Pandemic'. *Partecipazione e Conflitto* [Online] 15 (3): 697–719.

Mudde, Cas. 2007. *Populist Radical Right Parties in Europe*. Cambridge: Cambridge University Press. https://doi.org/10.1017/CBO9780511492037.

Murru, Maria Francesca. 2022. 'QAnon and Its Conspiracy Milieu: The Italian Case'. In *Populism and Science in Europe*, edited by Hande Eslen-Ziya and Alberta Giorgi, 163–84. London: Palgrave.

Nordheim, Gerret von, Jonas Rieger, and Katharina Kleinen-von Königslöw. 2021. 'From the Fringes to the Core—An Analysis of Right-Wing Populists' Linking Practices in Seven EU Parliaments and Switzerland'. *Digital Journalism*, September, 1–19. https://doi.org/10.1080/21670811.2021.1970602.

O'Toole, Roger. 1977. *The Precipitous Path: Studies in Political Sects*. Toronto: Peter Martin Associates.

Offe, Claus. 2011. 'What, If Anything, May We Mean by "Progressive Politics Today?"'. Rethinking Progress and Ensuring a Secure Future for All: What We Can Learn from the Crisis'. *Trends in Social Cohesion* 22: 79–92.

———. 2021. 'Corona Pandemic Policy: Exploratory Notes on Its "Epistemic Regime"'. In *Pandemics, Politics and Society: Critical Perspectives on the Covid-19 Crisis*, 25–42. Berlin: De Gruyter. https://doi.org/10.1515/9783110713350-003.

Pantenburg, Johannes, Sven Reichardt, and Benedikt Sepp. 2021. 'Wissensparallelwelten der »Querdenker«'. In *Die Corona-Proteste aus kultur- und sozialwissenschaftlicher Perspektive*, edited by Sven Reichardt, 29–66. Frankfurt: Campus Verlag. https://kops.uni-konstanz.de/handle/123456789/54271.

Parmigiani, Giovanna. 2021. 'Magic and Politics: Conspirituality and COVID-19'. *Journal of the American Academy of Religion* 89 (2): 506–29. https://doi.org/10.1093/jaarel/lfab053.

Paternotte, David, and Roman Kuhar. 2018. 'Disentangling and Locating the "Global Right": Anti-Gender Campaigns in Europe'. *Politics and Governance*, The Feminist Project under Threat in Europe 6 (3): 6–19.

Perrineau, Pascal. 1997. *Le Symptome Le Pen: Radiographie Des Electeurs Du Front National*. Espace Du Politique. Paris: Fayard.

Pilati, Federico, and Andrea Miconi. 2022. 'The "Green Pass" Controversy in the Italian Twittersphere: A Digital Methods Mapping'. *Partecipazione e Conflitto* [Online] 15 (3): 549–66.

Prearo, Massimo. 2020. *L'ipotesi neocattolica. Politologia dei movimenti anti-gender*. Quaderni di Teoria Critica della Società. Milano: Mimesis Edizioni. https://www.mimesisedizioni.it/libro/9788857570167.

Quarantelli, E. L., and R. R. Dynes. 1977. 'Response to Social Crisis and Disaster'. *Annual Review of Sociology* 3 (1): 23–49. https://doi.org/10.1146/annurev.so.03.080177.000323.

Rafael, Simone. 2021. 'Conspiracy Ideologies during the Pandemic: The Rise of QAnon in Europe'. *HOPE Not Hate*. https://hopenothate.org.uk/chapter/europeanstateofhate-the-rise-of-qanon/.

Rao, Hayagreeva, and Henrich R. Greve. 2017. 'Disasters and Community Resilience: Spanish Flu and the Formation of Retail Cooperatives in Norway'. *AMJ* 61: 5–25. https://doi.org/10.5465/amj.2016.0054.

Reich, Jennifer A. 2014. 'Neoliberal Mothering and Vaccine Refusal: Imagined Gated Communities and the Privilege of Choice'. *Gender & Society* 28 (5): 679–704. https://doi.org/10.1177/0891243214532711.

Reichardt, Sven. 2021. *Die Misstrauensgemeinschaft Der »Querdenker«: Die Corona-Proteste Aus Kultur- Und Sozialwissenschaftlicher Perspektive*. Frankfurt: Campus Verlag.

Reset. n.d. '"ViVi per Un Mondo Libero". Violent Italian Conspiracy Group Harasses Politicians and Spreads Vaccine Disinformation in Blatant Breach of Facebook Rules'. https://www.reset.tech/documents/italy-antivax-report.pdf.

Reuband, Karl-Heinz. 2021. 'Regionale AfD-Milieus und die Dynamik der Corona-Ausbreitung—Eine Analyse auf der Basis kreisfreier Städte und Landkreise in Sachsen'. *Zeitschrift für Parteienwissenschaften*, 1 (April): 1–14. https://doi.org/10.24338/mip-20211-14.

Richter, Christoph, and Axel Salheiser. 2021. 'Die Corona-Pandemie als Katalysator des Rechtsextremismus und Rechtspopulismus in Thüringen, Deutschland und Europa?' Institut für Demokratie und Zivilgesellschaft (IDZ). https://www.idz-jena.de/wsddet/wsd9–8.

Richter, Christoph, Maximilian Wächter, Jost Reinecke, Axel Salheiser, Matthias Quent, and Matthias Wjst. 2021. 'Politische Raumkultur als Verstärker der Corona-Pandemie? Einflussfaktoren auf die regionale Inzidenzentwicklung in Deutschland in der ersten und zweiten Pandemiewelle 2020'. *ZRex—Zeitschrift für Rechtsextremismusforschung* 1 (2). https://www.budrich-journals.de/index.php/zrex/article/view/38483.

Roberts, Kenneth M. 2015. *Changing Course in Latin America: Party Systems in the Neoliberal Era*. Cambridge Studies in Comparative Politics. New York: Cambridge University Press.

Rocke, Anja. 2021. *Soziologie Der Selbst-Optimierung*. Berlin: Suhrkamp.

Rohlinger, Deana A., and David S. Meyer. 2021. 'Protest During a Pandemic: How COVID-19 Affected Social Movements in the U.S'. SocArXiv. https://doi.org/10.31235/osf.io/qk25r.

Roose, Jochen. 2020. *Sie Sind Überall. Eine Repräsentative Umfrage Zu Verschwörungstheorien*. Berlin: Konrad-Adenauer-Stiftung. https://www.kas.de/documents/252038/7995358/Eine+repr%C3%A4sentative+Umfrage+zu+Verschw%C3%B6rungstheorien.pdf/0f422364-9ff1-b058-9b02-617e15f8bbd8?version=1.0&t=1599144843148.

Roozenbeek, Jon, Claudia R. Schneider, Sarah Dryhurst, John Kerr, Alexandra L. J. Freeman, Gabriel Recchia, Anne Marthe van der Bles, and Sander van der Linden. 2020. 'Susceptibility to Misinformation about COVID-19 around the World'. *Royal Society Open Science* 7 (10): 201199. https://doi.org/10.1098/rsos.201199.

Rosenberg, Charles E. 1989. 'What Is an Epidemic? AIDS in Historical Perspective'. *Daedalus* 118 (2): 1–17. https://www.jstor.org/stable/20025233.

Rucht, Dieter, and Thomas Ohlemacher. 1992. 'Protest Event Data: Collection, Uses and Perspectives'. In *Studying Collective Action*, edited by Mario Diani and Ron Eyerman, 76–106. London: Sage.

Sanders, Chris, and Kristin Burnett. 2019. 'The Neoliberal Roots of Modern Vaccine Hesitancy'. *Journal of Health and Social Sciences*. https://doi.org/10.19204/2019/thnl4.

Scheppele, Kim Lane. 2010. 'Exceptions That Prove the Rule: Embedding Emergency Government in Everyday Constitutional Life'. In *The Limits of Constitutional Democracy*, edited by Jeffrey K. Tulis and Stephen Macedo, 224–54. New Jersey: Princeton University Press.

Schließler, Clara, Nele Hellweg, and Oliver Decker. 2020. 'Aberglaube, Esoterik und Verschwörungsmentalität in Zeiten der Pandemie'. In *Autoritäre Dynamiken: Alte Ressentiments—neue Radikalität*, edited by Oliver Decker and Elmar Brähler, 1st edition, 283–308. Gießen: Verlag. https://doi.org/10.30820/9783837977714.

Smith, Philip J., Susan Y. Chu, and Lawrence E. Barker. 2004. 'Children Who Have Received No Vaccines: Who Are They and Where Do They Live?' *Pediatrics* 114 (1): 187–95. https://doi.org/10.1542/peds.114.1.187.

Snow, David. 2023. 'COVID-19, Collective Behaviour and Protest'. In *Encyclopaedia of Political and Social Movements*, edited by David Snow, Donatella della Porta, Doug McAdam, and Bert Klandermans, 2nd edition, 186–192. Oxford, UK: Blackwell Publishing Ltd.

Snow, David, Daniel Cress, Liam Downey, and Andrew Jones. 1998. 'Disrupting the "Quotidian": Reconceptualizing the Relationship Between Breakdown and the Emergence of Collective Action'. *Mobilization: An International Quarterly* 3 (1): 1–22. https://doi.org/10.17813/maiq.3.1.n41nv8m267572r30.

Snow, David A. 2013. 'Framing and Social Movements'. In *The Wiley-Blackwell Encyclopedia of Social and Political Movements*, edited by David A. Snow, Donatella della Porta, Bert Klandermans, and Doug McAdam, 470–475. Malden: Wiley-Blackwell John Wiley & Sons, Ltd. https://doi.org/10.1002/9780470674871.wbespm434.

Snow, David A., and Robert D. Benford. 1988. 'Ideology, Frame Resonance and Participant Mobilization'. *International Social Movement Research* 1: 197–217.

Snow, David A., and Colin Bernatzky. 2023. 'Anti-Vaccine Movement (United States)'. In *The Wiley Blackwell Encyclopedia of Political and Social Movements*, edited by Donatella Della Porta, David A. Snow, Doug McAdam, and Bert Klandermans, 2nd edition, 511–513. London: Blackwell.

Snow, David A., E. Burke Rochford, Steven K. Worden, and Robert D. Benford. 1986. 'Frame Alignment Processes, Micromobilization, and Movement Participation'. *American Sociological Review* 51 (4): 464–81. https://doi.org/10.2307/2095581.

Snowden, Frank M. 2020. *Epidemics and Society: From the Black Death to the Present*. Connecticut: Yale University Press.

Sol Hart, P., Sedona Chinn, and Stuart Soroka. 2020. 'Politicization and Polarization in COVID-19 News Coverage'. *Science Communication* 42 (5): 679–97. https://doi.org/10.1177/1075547020950735.

Song, Hoon. 2010. *Pigeon Trouble: Bestiary Biopolitics in a Deindustrialized America*. Philadelphia, PA: University of Pennsylvania Press.

Speit, Andreas. 2021. *Verqueres Denken. Gefährliche Weltbilder in Alternativen Milieus*. Berlin: Ch. Links Verlag.

Spöri, Tobias, and Jan Eichhorn. 2021. 'Wer Glaubt (Nicht Mehr) an Corona- Verschwörungsmythen?' https://infodienst.bzga.de/migration-flucht-und-gesundheit/materialien/wer-glaubt-an-corona-verschwoerungsmythen/

Staggenborg, Suzanne. 1993. 'Critical Events and the Mobilization of the Pro-Choice Movement'. *Research in Political Sociology* 6 (1): 319–45. https://doi.org/10.2307/800657.

Stavrakakis, Yannis, and Giorgos Katsambekis. 2020. 'Populism and the Pandemic: A Collaborative Report'. Report. Loughborough: Loughborough University. https://repository.lboro.ac.uk/articles/report/Populism_and_the_pandemic_A_collaborative_report/12546284/1.

Sutcliffe, Steven, J. 2003. *Children of the New Age: A History of Spiritual Practices*. New York: Routledge.

Swidler, Ann. 1986. 'Culture in Action: Symbols and Strategies'. *American Sociological Review* 51 (2): 273–86. https://doi.org/10.2307/2095521.

Taggart, Paul. 1995. 'New Populist Parties in Western Europe'. *West European Politics* 18 (1): 34–51. https://doi.org/10.1080/01402389508425056.

Taggart, Paul A. 2000. *Populism*. Maidenhead: Open University Press.

Tarrow, Sidney. 1994. *Power in Movement: Social Movements and Contentious Politics*, 2nd edition. Cambridge Studies in Comparative Politics. Cambridge: Cambridge University Press. https://doi.org/10.1017/CBO9780511813245.

Teune, Simon. 2021. 'Querdenken Und Die Bewegungsforschung—Neue Herausforderung Oder Déjà-Vu?' *Forschungsjournal Soziale Bewegungen* 34 (2): 326–34. https://doi.org/10. 1515/fjsb-2021-0029.

Tierney, Kathleen. 2019. *Disasters: A Sociological Approach*. Cambridge: Polity.

Tilly, Charles. 1992. 'Where Do Rights Come From?' In *Contributions to the Comparative Politics of Development*, edited by Lars Mjoset, 9–37. Oslo: Institute for Social Research.

———. 2003. *The Politics of Collective Violence*. Cambridge Studies in Contentious Politics. Cambridge: Cambridge University Press. https://doi.org/10.1017/CBO9780511819131.

Turner, Bryan, S. 2021. 'The Political Theology of Covid-19: A Comparative History of Human Responses to Catastrophes'. In *Pandemics, Politics and Society: Critical Perspectives on the Covid-19 Crisis*, edited by Gerard Delanty, 139–56. Berlin: De Gruyter.

Vandenberghe, Frédéric, and Jean-François Véran. 2021. 'The Pandemic as a Global Social Total Fact'. In *Critical Perspectives on the Covid-19 Crisis*, edited by Gerard Delanty, 171–88. Berlin, Boston: De Gruyter. https://doi.org/doi:10.1515/9783110713350-012.

Vieten, Ulrike M. 2020. 'The "New Normal" and "Pandemic Populism": The COVID-19 Crisis and Anti-Hygienic Mobilisation of the Far-Right'. *Social Sciences* 9 (9): 165. https://doi.org/ 10.3390/socsci9090165.

Virchow, Fabian, and Alexander Häusler. 2020. 'Pandemie-Leugnung Und Extreme Rechte in Nordrhein-Westfalen'. BICC—Bonn International Centre for Conflict Studies. November 2020. https://www.bicc.de/publications/publicationpage/publication/pandemie-leugnung-und-extreme-rechte-in-nordrhein-westfalen–1019/.

Weiß, Volker,. 2021. 'Gemeinsam Gegen Den "Great Reset" Synergien Zwischen Neuer Rechter Und Corona-Protesten'. Edited by Wolfgang Benz *Querdenken. Protestbewegung Zwischen Demokratieverachtung, Hass und Aufruhr*, 214–30. Berlin: Metropol Verlag.

Vraga, Emily, Teresa Myers, John Kotcher, Lindsey Beall, and Ed Maibach. 2018. 'Scientific Risk Communication about Controversial Issues Influences Public Perceptions of Scientists' Political Orientations and Credibility'. *Royal Society Open Science* 5 (2): 170505. https://doi. org/10.1098/rsos.170505.

Ward, Charlotte, and David Voas. 2011. 'The Emergence of Conspirituality'. *Institute for Social and Economic Research (ISER)* 26: 103–21. http://dx.doi.org/10.1080/13537903.2011. 539846.

Ward, Jeremy, K. 2016. 'Rethinking the Antivaccine Movement Concept: A Case Study of Public Criticism of the Swine Flu Vaccine's Safety in France'. *Social Science & Medicine* 159: 48–57 https://doi.org/10.1016/j.socscimed.2016.05.003.

Watkins, Susan. 2020. 'Politics and Pandemics'. *New Left Review* 125 (October): 5–17.

Wetzel, Juliane. 2021. 'Antisemitismus—Bindekitt Für Verdrossene Und Verweigerer'. In *Querdenken. Protestbewegung Zwischen Demokratieverachtung, Hass und Aufruhr*, edited by Wolfgang Benz, 55–75. Berlin: Metropol Verlag.

White, Jonathan. 2019. *Politics of Last Resort: Governing by Emergency in the European Union*. Oxford: Oxford University Press.

———. 2021. 'Emergency Europe after Covid-19'. In *Pandemics, Politics, and Society: Critical Perspectives on the Covid-19 Crisis*, edited by Gerard Delanty, 75–92. Berlin: De Gruyter.

Williams, Rhys H. 2004. 'The Cultural Contexts of Collective Action: Constraints, Opportunities, and the Symbolic Life of Social Movements'. In *The Blackwell Companion to Social Movements*, edited by David A. Snow, Sarah A. Soule, Hanspeter Kriesi, and Holly J. McCammon, 91–115. New Jersey: John Wiley & Sons. https://doi.org/10.1002/ 9780470999103.ch5.

Wissenschaft im Dialog. 2020. 'Wissenschaftsbarometer 2020'. https://www.wissenschaft-im-dialog.de/projekte/wissenschaftsbarometer/wissenschaftsbarometer-2020/.

Wissenschaft im Dialog. 2021. 'Science Barometer'.

Wodak, Ruth. 2015. *The Politics of Fear: What Right-Wing Populist Discourses Mean.* London: SAGE publications. https://doi.org/10.4135/9781446270073.

———. 2019. 'The Trajectory of Far-Right Populism—A Discourse-Analytical Perspective'. In *The Far Right and the Environment*, 21–37. Routledge. https://doi.org/10.4324/9781351104043-2.

Wondreys, Jakub, and Cas Mudde. 2022. 'Victims of the Pandemic? European Far-Right Parties and COVID-19'. *Nationalities Papers* 50 (1): 86–103. https://doi.org/10.1017/nps.2020.93.

World Health Organization, Regional Office for South-East Asia. 2020. 'Communicating and Managing Uncertainty in the COVID-19 Pandemic: A Quick Guide'. https://www.who.int/docs/default-source/searo/whe/coronavirus19/managing-uncertainty-in-covid-19-a-quick-guide.pdf.

Ylä-Anttila, Tuukka. 2018. "Populist knowledge: 'Post-truth' repertoires of contesting epistemic authorities." *European Journal of Cultural and Political Sociology* 5: 356–388.

York, Michael. 1995. *The Emerging Network: A Sociology of the New Age and Neo-Pagan Movements.* Maryland: Rowman & Littlefield.

———. 2001. 'New Age Commodification and Appropriation of Spirituality'. *Journal of Contemporary Religion* 16 (3): 361–72. https://doi.org/10.1080/13537900120077177.

Ypi, Lea. 2012. *Global Justice and Avant-Garde Political Agency.* Oxford: Oxford University Press.

Online sources

All documents last accessed 30 October 2022.

Agamben, Giorgio. 2021a. 'La nuda vita e il vaccino'. Quodlibet (blog). 16 April 2021. https://www.quodlibet.it/giorgio-agamben-la-nuda-vita-e-il-vaccino.

———. 2021b. 'Cittadini di seconda classe'. Quodlibet (blog). 16 July 2021. https://www.quodlibet.it/giorgio-agamben-cittadini-di-seconda-classe.

———. 2021c. 'Una comunità nella società'. Quodlibet (blog). 17 September 2021. https://www.quodlibet.it/giorgio-agamben-una-comunit-14-ella-societa.

Ancora Italia Palermo. n.d. 'Manifesto'. Ancora Italia Palermo (blog). https://www.ancoraitaliapalermo.it/manifesto/.

ANSA, Agenzia. 2021. 'Trieste, perché protestano i portuali e chi è Stefano Puzzer—Cronaca'. *Agenzia ANSA*, 18 October 2021, sec. Cronaca. https://www.ansa.it/sito/notizie/cronaca/2021/10/18/dopo-la-protesta-al-porto-trieste-e-la-capitale-no-pass-e-puzzer-suo-leader_1217f1ce-54e6-46bd-81bc-a50efcdfa54e.html.

AsSIS. 2022. 'Green-pass e obblighi vaccinali per covid non hanno fondamento scientifico, e che queste politiche, proprio alla luce delle prove disponibili, andrebbero riviste subito'. AsSIS (blog). 27 January 2022. https://www.assis.it/green-pass-e-obblighi-vaccinali-per-covid-non-hanno-fondamento/.

AttoPrimo. 2021. 'Appello dei docenti universitari: "No al Green Pass"'. AttoPrimo ODV (blog). 12 September 2021. https://www.attoprimo.org/appello-dei-docenti-universitari-no-al-green-pass/.

AttoPrimo ODV. 2021. 'Coordinamento 15 ottobre'. AttoPrimo ODV (blog). 27 December 2021. https://www.attoprimo.org/coordinamento-15-ottobre/.

Becchi, Franz. 2021. '"Diritti fonamentali sono ormai diventati semplice concessioni", la denuncia di preterossi'. ByoBlu—La TV dei Cittadini (blog). 15 November 2021. https://www.byoblu.com/2021/11/15/geminello-preterossi-diritti-sono-concessioni/.

———. 2022. '"Fermiamo subito la vaccinazione di massa", l'appello del nobel Montagnier. Cambiano tutte le carte in gioco? ByoBlu—La TV dei Cittadini (blog). 15 January 2022. https://www.byoblu.com/2022/01/15/luc-montagnier-fermiamo-subito-vaccinazione-di-massa/.

Bianco, Filippo, and Gaetano Rotondo. 2021. '#NO GREEN PASS'. Comitato Liberi Pensatori (blog). 16 September 2021. https://comitatoliberipensatori.com/no-green-pass/.

Bocci, Michele. 2019. 'Vaccini a scuola, fronda M5S: "No all'emendamento, l'obbligo serve"'. la Repubblica, 1 April 2019. https://www.repubblica.it/salute/medicina-e-ricerca/2019/04/01/news/vaccini_no_all_emendamento_l_obbligo_serve_-223017939/.

Bufale. 2022. 'La Procura archivia le denunce contro Draghi e i novax la prendono male: interviene la DIGOS'. Bufale (blog). 7 February 2022. https://www.bufale.net/la-procura-archivia-le-minacce-contro-draghi-e-i-novax-la-prendono-male-interviene-la-digos/.

Catania Creattiva. 2022. 'Il Premio Nobel Michael Levitt Sul Covid: "Il Livello Di Stupidità Raggiunto è Pazzesco"'. Catania CreAttiva Blog & Web Radio/TV, 20 January 2022. https://cataniacreattiva.it/il-premio-nobel-michael-levitt-sul-covid-il-livello-di-stupidita-raggiunto-e-pazzesco/.

C.I.A.T.D.M., Coordinamento 15 Ottobre, Associazione ContiamoCi!, e l'Associazione di Studi e Informazione sulla Salute (AsSIS), and a seguito delle richieste della Commissione Medico-Scientifica Indipendente (CMSi). 2022. 'Comunicato Stampa 11_1_22'.

Comilva. n.d. 'Chi Siamo | Comilva'. https://www.comilva.org/lassociazione/chi-siamo.

Comitato Liberi Pensatori. n.d. 'Benvenuto'. Comitato Liberi Pensatori (blog). https://comitatoliberipensatori.com/.

Coordinamento Istruzione per la Libertà. 2022. 'Il nostro intervento il 15 gennaio a Roma'. Coordinamento Istruzione per la Libertà (blog). 19 January 2022. https://cilperlaliberta.wordpress.com/2022/01/19/il-nostro-intervento-il-15-gennaio-a-roma/.

Coordinamento 15 Ottobre. 2021. Il volantinaggio della 'consapevolezza'. https://www.coordinamento15ottobre.it/materiale-volantinaggio/

Coordinamento 15 Ottobre. 2022. 'Comunicato Stampa: Pandemia, Vaccini e Restrizioni'. Coordinamento 15 Ottobre, January. chrome-extension://efaidnbmnnnibpcajpcglclefindmkaj/https://www.attoprimo.org/wp-content/uploads/2022/01/Comunicato-Stampa-11_1_22.pdf (accessed 30 October 2022).

Coordinamento 15 ottobre. n.d. 'Coordinamento 15 Ottobre'. https://www.coordinamento15ottobre.it/?fbclid=IwAR1LcQqsqSqmT3xc2XTL4-AWwkC7nrx5ecKXn7t-boJK3eT_Nr7loQpaFt4.

COSPASIR. Comitato parlamentare per la sicurezza della Repubblica (2021) Doc. XXXIV n. 8., Senato della Repubblica, https://www.senato.it/leg/18/BGT/Schede/docnonleg/44158.htm.

Crimaldi, Giuseppe. 2022. 'No vax, tensioni al tribunale di Napoli: "Siamo pronti a denunciare Draghi"'. Il Mattino, 29 January 2022. https://www.ilmattino.it/napoli/cronaca/no_vax_tribunale_di_napoli_ultime_notizie_oggi-6469126.html.

Difendersi Ora. n.d. 'Chi siamo'. Difendersi Ora. https://www.difendersiora.it/chi-siamo.

Dipartimento Giuridico Generazioni Future. 2021. 'Sulle misure "di contenimento dell'epidemia" adottate dal Governo il 29/12/21'. Generazioni Future (blog). 31 December 2021. https://generazionifuture.org/sulle-misure-di-contenimento-dellepidemia-adottate-dal-governo-il-29-12-21/.

———. 2022. 'Commissione DuPre—nota del 2 gennaio 2022'. Generazioni Future (blog). 2 January 2022. https://generazionifuture.org/commissione-dupre-nota-del-2-gennaio-2022/.

Fagnani, Giovanna Maria. 2022. 'Milano, Prof (No Vax) sospeso e senza stipendio in sciopero della fame davanti all'ingresso della Scuola'. Corriere Della Sera, 7 February 2022. https://milano.corriere.it/notizie/cronaca/22_febbraio_07/milano-prof-no-vax-sospeso-senza-stipendio-sciopero-fame-all-ingresso-scuola-af980286-87fa-11ec-8804-7df4f9fb61d8.shtml.

Famà, Irene. 2022. 'L'appello su Telegram dei No Vax: "Dar fuoco alla procura di Torino"'. La Stampa, 7 February 2022. https://www.lastampa.it/torino/2022/02/07/news/l_appello_su_telegram_dei_no_vax_dar_fuoco_a_procura_torino_-2849795/.

Franceschini, Massimo. 2021a. 'L'inettitudine politica ci costringerà sulla strada'. Attivismo.info (blog). 30 November 2021. https://www.attivismo.info/linettitudine-politica-ci-costringera-sulla-strada/.

———. 2021b. 'Il coraggio di dire basta ed agire politicamente'. massimo franceschini blog (blog). 29 December 2021. https://www.massimofranceschiniblog.it/2021/12/29/il-coraggio-di-dire-basta-ed-agire-politicamente/.

Fronte del Dissenso. 2021. 'Scopi e funzionamento del fronte del dissenso'. www.sollevazione.it/2021/10/scopi-e-funzionamento-del-fronte-del-dissenso.html

Generazioni Future. 2021a. 'Giorgio Agamben: Sulla democrazia'. Generazioni Future (blog). 28 December 2021. https://generazionifuture.org/giorgio-agamben-interventi/.

———. 2021b. 'Sulle misure "di contenimento dell'epidemia" adottate dal Governo il 29/12/21'. Generazioni Future (blog). 31 December 2021. https://generazionifuture.org/sulle-misure-di-contenimento-dellepidemia-adottate-dal-governo-il-29-12-21/.

———. 2022a. 'Manifesto per la dichiarazione di emergenza giuridica'. Generazioni Future (blog). 9 January 2022. https://generazionifuture.org/manifesto-per-la-dichiarazione-di-emergenza-giuridica/.

———. 2022b. 'Replica Costruttiva e Invito al Dialogo del Dipartimento Giuridico di Generazioni Future'. Generazioni Future (blog). 13 January 2022. https://generazionifuture.org/replica-costruttiva-e-invito-al-dialogo-del-dipartimento-giuridico-di-generazioni-future/.

Gentile, Gustavo. 2022. 'Nuove minacce No-Vax su Telegram a Draghi e Bassetti'. Cronache della Campania (blog). 16 February 2022. https://www.cronachedellacampania.it/2022/02/minacce-no-vax-su-telegram/.

Giannoli, Viola. 2022. 'Divise di deportati e volantini sulla Shoah, l'ultimo oltraggio dei No Vax nel Giorno della Memoria'. la Repubblica, 27 January 2022. https://www.repubblica.it/cronaca/2022/01/27/news/divise_di_deportati_e_volantini_sulla_shoah_l_ultimo_oltraggio_dei_no_vax_nel_giorno_della_memoria-335467807/.

Gioia, Emiliano. 2021. '#DisdettaAdesso!' Il blog di SìAMO (blog). 13 October 2021. https://www.movimentosiamo.it/blog/2021/10/13/disdettaadesso/.

Giulia. 2022. '"Abbiamo calpestato la scienza". Spopola sui social l'intervento del Prof. Perrone al Parlamento europeo'. Il Paragone, 21 January 2022. https://www.ilparagone.it/interventi/abbiamo-calpestato-la-scienza-spopola-sui-social-lintervento-del-prof-perrone-al-parlamento-europeo/.

Goccia. 2021. 'Appello al Governo per l'esenzione dal green pass per gli studenti che utilizzano mezzi di trasporto pubblici'. Gruppo 'Goccia a goccia' (blog). 30 November 2021. https://gocciaagoccia.net/2021/11/30/appello-al-governo-per-lesenzione-dal-green-pass-per-gli-studenti-che-utilizzano-mezzi-di-trasporto-pubblici/.

———. 2022. 'Cosa è Andato Storto Nelle Politiche Anti-COVID'. Gruppo 'Goccia a goccia' (blog). 19 July 2022. https://gocciaagoccia.net/author/disaragliamici1673/.

Goyal, Rishi, Arden Hegele, and Dennis Tenen. 2021. 'Op-Ed: How "My Body, My Choice" Came to Define the Vaccine Skepticism Movement'. Los Angeles Times, 22 May 2021. https://www.latimes.com/opinion/story/2021-05-22/vaccine-hesitancy-language-covid.

Gruppo Salute. 2020. 'Io Non Mi Vaccino Perché'. Movimento 3V Partito Poltiico (blog). 29 December 2020. https://www.movimento3v.it/io-non-mi-vaccino-perche/.

HuffPost Italia. 2021. 'No Vax in piazza contro il green pass, manifestazioni in 80 città'. HuffPost Italia, 24 July 2021. https://www.huffingtonpost.it/entry/no-vax-in-piazza-contro-il-green-pass-manifestazioni-in-80-citta_it_60fbfee4e4b0a807eeb23cf9/.

———. 2022. 'A Bari i no vax in fila davanti alla caserma: "Denunciamo Draghi per il ricatto del Green Pass"'. HuffPost Italia, 2 February 2022. https://www.huffingtonpost.it/covid/2022/02/02/news/bari_no_vax_denuncia–8642697/.

il Dolomiti. 2021. 'Sciopero della fame dei vigili del fuoco no vax contro il green pass: "Introdurremo liquidi onde evitare complicanze mediche"'. il Dolomiti, 3 November 2021. https://www.ildolomiti.it/cronaca/2021/sciopero-della-fame-dei-vigili-del-fuoco-no-vax-contro-il-green-pass-introdurremo-liquidi-onde-evitare-complicanze-mediche.

Il Fatto Quotidiano. 2021. 'Assalto alla Cgil, altre 6 misure cautelari: sono militanti di Forza Nuova e dei movimenti No Vax'. Il Fatto Quotidiano, 30 October 2021. https://www.ilfattoquotidiano.it/2021/10/30/assalto-alla-cgil-eseguite-altre-sei-misure-cautelari-anche-il-leader-veronese-di-forza-nuova/6374015/.

Il Gazzettino. 2022. 'Maestra assunta il lunedì e licenziata il martedì, per 15 volte. E non ha visto un centesimo: la decisione del Tar'. Il Gazzettino, 12 February 2022. https://www.ilgazzettino.it/nordest/treviso/maestra_contratto_scuola_supplenze_temporanee_part_time-6499653.html.

Il Reggino. 2021. 'Reggio, il Codacons denuncia Draghi, Conte e Speranza · Il Reggino', 29 September 2021. https://www.ilreggino.it/cronaca/2021/09/29/reggio-il-codacons-denuncia-draghi-conte-e-speranza/.

Il Tempo.it. 2022. 'Il prof no-vax Tutino fa lo sciopero della fame e ottiene l'esenzione dal vaccino', 13 January 2022. https://www.iltempo.it/politica/2022/01/13/news/davide-tutino-sciopero-fame-contro-vaccino-green-pass-esenzione-no-vax-obbligo-governo-draghi-covid–30086238/.

Istanza diritti umani IDU. n.d. 'Campagna Informativa Libertà Di Cura. Gofundme.Com. https://www.gofundme.com/f/campagna-informativa-libert-di-cura.

Iozzoli, Giovanni. 2021. 'Immunizzati alla democrazia'. Carmilla online (blog). 8 October 2021. https://www.carmillaonline.com/2021/10/08/immunizzati-alla-democrazia/.

La Fionda. n.d. 'Manifesto—La Fionda'. https://www.lafionda.com/manifesto/.

La Nazione. 2021. 'Prof sospesi in presidio davanti alle scuole. "Aspettiamo il ritorno della democrazia"—Cronaca'. La Nazione, 22 December 2021. https://www.lanazione.it/firenze/cronaca/prof-sospesi-non-vaccinati-presidio-scuole-1.7177884.

Lazzaretti, Giovanni. 2021. 'Il Covid Ed Il Generale Autunno—Attivismo.Info'. Attivismo.Info (blog). 7 November 2021. https://www.attivismo.info/il-covid-ed-il-generale-autunno/.

Liberiamo l'Italia. 2021. 'Tesi sul cybercapitalismo'. Liberiamo l'Italia (blog). 16 November 2021. https://www.liberiamolitalia.org/tesi-sul-cybercapitalismo (accessed 30 October 2022).

Liberiamo l'Italia. 2022. 'Aderisci a Liberiamo L'Italia'. Liberiamo l'Italia, 28 January 2022. https://www.liberiamolitalia.org/2022/01/28/aderisci-a-liberiamo-litalia/ (accessed 30 October 2022).

———. n.d. 'Appello Manifestazione 12 Ottobre 2019'. Liberiamo l'Italia (blog). https://www.liberiamolitalia.org/firma-lappellofirma-lappello-liberiamo-litalia-manifestazione-12-ottobre.

Lorenzo. 2022. 'Blitz di CasaPound e Movimento Nazionale in alcuni luoghi simbolo di Milano per lanciare un messaggio: difendiamo la nostra città!' CasaPound Italia (blog). 17 January 2022. https://www.casapounditalia.org/blitz-di-casapound-e-movimento-nazionale-in-alcuni-luoghi-simbolo-di-milano-per-lanciare-un-messaggio-difendiamo-la-nostra-citta/.

Luna Rossa. 2021. 'Il Coordinamento dei Lavoratori Portuali di Trieste …'. Nuova resistenza antifa (blog). 15 October 2021. https://www.nuovaresistenza.org/2021/10/il-coordinamento-dei-lavoratori-portuali-di-trieste/.

Maccentelli, Nico. 2022. 'Collettivismo… forzato?' Carmilla on line (blog). 18 January 2022. https://www.carmillaonline.com/2022/01/18/collettivismo-forzato/.

Mauro, Marco di. 2022. 'Piovono denunce su Draghi da tutta Italia'. Come Don Chisciotte (blog). 28 January 2022. https://comedonchisciotte.org/piovono-denunce-su-draghi-da-tutta-italia/.

Miceli, Jacopo di. 2021. 'Manifestazione Green Pass Torino #NoGreenPass, La Stampa—No Psico #Dittatura / 7 Agosto 2021'. 12 August 2021. https://www.youtube.com/watch?v=yLNanVtwTX8.

Morandi, Francesca. 2022. 'Querela contro Draghi e il Governo, il Movimento Fortitudo davanti al Tribunale'. La Provincia Cremona, 3 February 2022. https://www.laprovinciacr.it/video/cronaca/377655/querela-contro-draghi-il-movimento-fortitudo-davanti-al-tribunale.html.

Movimento Io Apro. 2021. 'Statuto'. Movimento Io Apro. https://www.movimentoioapro.com/wp-content/uploads/2021/11/Statuto-IoApro.pdf (accessed 30 October 2022).

Movimento 3V. 2022. 'Obbligo vaccinale: come resistere'. 20 January 2022. https://www.movimento3v.it/obbligo-vaccinale-come-resistere/.

Movimento IoApro. n.d. a 'Statuto—Movimento IoApro'. https://www.movimentoioapro.com/istruzione/.

———. n.d.b 'L'Italia che prospera'. https://www.movimentoioapro.com/.

News Prima. 2022. 'L'ultima trovata No vax: denunciano Draghi e il Governo per ricatto vaccinale. Il modulo nelle chat', 18 January 2022. https://newsprima.it/glocal-news/lultima-trovata-no-vax-denunciano-draghi-e-il-governo-per-ricatto-vaccinale-il-modulo-nelle-chat/.

nextQuotidiano. 2022. 'La mappa dei no green pass che aiuta, a loro insaputa, le forze dell'ordine a chiudere i locali che non chiedono la certificazione'. nextQuotidiano, 16 February 2022. https://www.nextquotidiano.it/ristoranti-no-green-pass-mappa-chiusura-polizia/.

Open. 2021a. 'No vax e No Green pass tornano in piazza. A Roma e Milano centinaia di persone—Foto e video'. Open, 11 September 2021. https://www.open.online/2021/09/11/covid-19-manifestazioni-no-green-pass-no-vax-roma-milano/.

———. 2021b. 'Dai vaccini «acqua sporca» al complotto mondiale, le teorie più strambe diffuse agli Stati generali dei No Green pass'. Open, 9 December 2021. https://www.open.online/2021/12/09/covid-19-stati-generali-no-green-pass-complotti/.

ParmaToday. 2022. 'Parmigiani no vax in coda davanti alla caserma per denunciare Draghi'. ParmaToday, 14 February 2022. https://www.parmatoday.it/attualita/no-vax-denunce-draghi-carabinieri.html.

'Partito Libertario | Facebook'. 2022. 22 January 2022. https://www.facebook.com/profile.php?id=100068761900654.

Pasquinelli, Moreno. 2021. 'Agamben o La Fuga Dal Mondo'. Sinistrainrete (blog). 30 December 2021. https://www.sinistrainrete.info/teoria/21928-moreno-pasquinelli-agamben-o-la-fuga-dal-mondo.html.

Polizia di Stato. 2021. 'Operazione "Basta Dittatura"'. 15 November 2021. https://www.poliziadistato.it/articolo/154361efa7c3148a6587974935.

Porro, Nicola. 2022. 'Super green pass e obbligo vaccinale, Draghi e Speranza citati in giudizio'. Nicola Porro (blog). 7 January 2022. https://www.nicolaporro.it/super-green-pass-e-obbligo-vaccinale-draghi-e-speranza-citati-in-giudizio/.

Prima Monza. 2022. 'Dodici in sciopero della fame contro il green pass'. Prima Monza, 2 March 2022. https://primamonza.it/attualita/dodici-in-sciopero-della-fame-contro-il-green-pass/.

R2020. 2021. '31 dicembre 2021: Usciamo dal Sistema! E tanti auguri a tutti …'. R2020 (blog). 27 December 2021. https://r2020.info/2021/12/27/31-dicembre-2021-usciamo-dal-sistema/.

———. n.d. 'Chi siamo'. *R2020* (blog). https://r2020.info/chi-siamo/.

Rec News. 2022. 'Covid, fioccano denunce e querele per Draghi e per Figliuolo'. Rec News, 19 January 2022. https://www.recnews.it/2022/01/19/rec-news-dir-zaira-bartucca-covid-fioccano-denunce-e-querele-per-draghi-e-per-figliuolo/.

Rovelli, Michela. 2017. 'Il blog ByoBlu e i 200 siti a cui Google ha tolto la pubblicità per la lotta alle fake news'. Corriere della Sera, 30 January 2017. http://www.corriere.it/tecnologia/cyber-cultura/cards/blog-byoblu-200-siti-cui-google-ha-tolto-pubblicita-la-lotta-fake-news/caso-byoblu_principale.shtml.

Sartori, Andrea. 2022. 'La "character assassination" di Benedetto XVI. In vista del conclave?' Visione TV, 21 January 2022. https://visionetv.it/la-character-assassination-di-benedetto-xvi-in-vista-del-conclave/.

Scott, Mark. 2020. 'QAnon Goes European'. *POLITICO* (blog). 23 October 2020. https://www.politico.eu/article/qanon-europe-coronavirus-protests/.

Sellner, Martin. 2020. 'Sellners Revolution- Alle an Einem Strang!' Compact. 24 May 2020. https://www.compact-online.de/sellners-revolution-_-alle-an-einem-strang/.

Sky TG24. 2020a. 'Napoli, proteste e scontri in piazza dopo le chiusure notturne. FOTO'. Sky TG24, 24 October 2020. https://tg24.sky.it/cronaca/2020/10/24/proteste-napoli-chiusure-covid.

———. 2020b. 'Firenze, corteo non autorizzato contro il Dpcm. Arresti e denunce', 31 October 2020. https://tg24.sky.it/cronaca/2020/10/30/firenze-manifestazione-anti-dpcm-cariche.

Spica, Giusi. 2022. 'Covid, morto Il biologo No Vax Franco Trinca'. la Repubblica, 4 February 2022. https://www.repubblica.it/cronaca/2022/02/04/news/covid_morto_il_biologo_no_vax_franco_trinca-336483960/.

Stach, Sabine, and Greta Hartmann. 2020. 'Friedliche Revolution 2.0? Zur Performativen Aneignung von 1989 Durch "Querdenken" Am 7. November 2020 in Leipzig'. Zeitgeschichte Online (blog). 23 November 2020. https://zeitgeschichte-online.de/geschichtskultur/friedliche-revolution-20.

Studenti contro il Green Pass. 2021. 'La lettera degli Studenti di Bergamo'. 15 September 2021. https://www.studenticontroilgreenpass.it/2021/09/15/la-lettera-degli-studenti-di-bergamo/.

———. 2022a. 'Sulla mia ex e su quel che accade'. 8 February 2022. https://www.studenticontroilgreenpass.it/2022/02/08/sulla-mia-ex-e-su-quel-che-accade2/.

———. 2022b. 'Uno a zero: palla al centro'. 8 February 2022. https://www.studenticontroilgreenpass.it/2022/02/08/uno-a-zero-palla-al-centro/.

Terra Nuova. 2022. 'Commissione Du.Pre: «È Un Dovere Difendere Lo Stato Costituzionale»'. TerraNuova. 3 January 2022. https://www.terranuova.it/News/Attualita/Commissione-Du.Pre-E-un-dovere-difendere-lo-Stato-costituzionale.

Timpano, Cinzia. 2022. 'Green Pass: 10 giorni di sciopero della fame contro le discrim-inazioni'. 24 February 2022. https://www.gazzettamatin.com/2022/02/24/green-pass-10-giorni-di-sciopero-della-fame-contro-le-discriminazioni/.

Tribuna di Treviso. 2022. 'Coda in tribunale a Treviso: sono i no-vax che vanno a denunciare Mario Draghi', 31 January 2022. https://mattinopadova.gelocal.it/regione/2022/01/31/news/coda-in-tribunale-a-treviso-sono-i-no-vax-che-vanno-a-denunciare-mario-draghi-1.41185920.

Vighi, Fabio. 2021. 'Paradigma Covid: collasso sistemico e fantasma pandemico'. La Fionda (blog). 22 June 2021. https://www.lafionda.org/2021/06/22/paradigma-covid-collasso-sistemico-e-fantasma-pandemico/.

———. 2022. 'In diretta da Milano: Uniti per la salvarci dalla dittatura sanitaria'. https://visionetv.it/in-diretta-da-milano-uniti-per-la-salvarci-dalla-dittatura-sanitaria/.

Visione TV. n.d. 'Visione TV'. https://visionetv.it/.

Zhok, Andrea. 2021a. 'Moralismo Vaccinale e Pruriti Totalitari, l'analisi Di Andrea Zhok—Il Paragone'. Il Paragone (blog). 28 July 2021. https://www.ilparagone.it/attualita/moralismo-vaccinale-e-pruriti-totalitari-lanalisi-di-andrea-zhok/.

———. 2021b. 'Sulla coercizione liberale'. controinformazione.info (blog). 7 August 2021. https://www.controinformazione.info/sulla-coercizione-liberale/.

———. 2021c. 'Per quanto possibile Buon Natale'. L'antidiplomatico. 24 December 2021. https://www.lantidiplomatico.it/dettnews-andrea__zhok__per_quanto_possibile_buon_natale/39602_44519/.

———. 2021d. 'Andrea Zhok - Sulla lettera di Cacciari e Agamben'. OP-ED, L'Antidiplomatico (lantidiplomatico.it). https://www.lantidiplomatico.it/dettnews-andrea_zhok__sulla_lettera_di_cacciari_e_agamben/39602_42472/.

———. 2022a. 'Cosa Possiamo Fare?' 8 January 2022. https://www.sinistrainrete.info/politica-italiana/21994-andrea-zhok-cosa-possiamo-fare.html.

———. 2022b. 'Infodemia Istituzionale e Stati Ontologici Dissociativi'. IdeeAzione (blog). 14 January 2022. https://www.ideeazione.com/infodemia-istituzionale-e-stati-ontologici-dissociativi/.

Index